Transition with Dignity

Sarah M. Hart

Transition with Dignity

School Leaving from the Perspectives of Young
Adults with Significant Disabilities

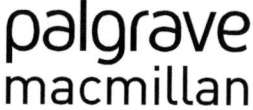

Sarah M. Hart 🆔
College of Education, Nursing, and Health Profession
University of Hartford
West Hartford, CT, USA

ISBN 978-981-97-2353-9   ISBN 978-981-97-2351-5   (eBook)
https://doi.org/10.1007/978-981-97-2351-5

This Palgrave Macmillan imprint is published by the registered company Springer Nature
Singapore Pte Ltd.
The registered company address is: 152 Beach Road, #21-01/04 Gateway East, Singapore
189721, Singapore

Paper in this product is recyclable.

Foreword 1

It takes a village to raise a child. He kainga hei whakatipu tamariki. We all need the guidance and support of a village on our journeys through life's changes and stages. While that need is common to us all, for some of us, transitions require intense planning, direction, and delivery.

With diagnoses of severe vision impairment, autism, and intellectual disability, my twin sons have never been able to contribute to the goalsetting or planning process of their education programmes. The goals we set while the twins were in school were small, and based on gaining independence and communication. All the decision-making ultimately rests with me. I measure each success and failure on their reactions, interactions, and participation.

They have experienced many transitions. From birth to diagnoses, to early childhood education, and through school (age 5–21 years). These transitions needed the input and guidance from many specialists, therapists, and educators from multiple agencies, alongside the family. All of us united in our efforts to support the twins to grow and develop into adulthood. As a consequence, our village grew ever bigger.

Transition to adult services for my sons was not the continuation of the school experience they had as young adults. Instead, the expectation was to join the group and work within a system that didn't meet their very individualized needs. For example, the twins did not have time to acclimate to new environments since visits were subject to staff availability. This would have allowed them and staff time to build relationships and for the family to build a rapport with new services.

As adults, enrollment in adult service centres is optional and funded through the social services government agency. The twins struggled to adapt to a new programme (set within an adapted open plan warehouse). It had no escape from the noise and activity of their peers. The expectation for them to join in resulted in the twins using behaviour to communicate their anxiety and need for space. This led to them being removed from activities to instead be taken for walks around the block, isolating them from the group. The plan was not working. This was evident not just in how their programme was run, but in the language used, with phrases like "we cannot cater for," "his noise is disturbing others," "he would be better off working from home," and of course, "we don't fund that" ... as just a few examples. It was advised my best (if not only) option was to run a programme from home, supported with funding administered by a service provider whose only involvement is the management of funds that they allocate to me quarterly.

Needless to say, it has been a journey of hits, misses, and resets. It is my opinion that for those young adults with extreme high needs the transition to adult services needs to happen earlier than age 20. Giving young adults choices and chances to develop within a new system or the option of trialing a service before committing to enrollment. These days, with the twins now at 31 years old, the village is small. Yet the loss to them and our family of the supportive village of school days is still raw.

Tāmaki Makaurau Auckland   Trish Lundon
Aotearoa, New Zealand
October 2023

Foreword 2

Every person goes through multiple transitions in a lifetime. Some may be seamless and some may require more planning and effort than others. There are natural transitions that occur when we enter a different stage in life—birthdays or milestones such as getting a driver's license or graduation. Many people successfully handle these types of transitions on their own while some may need a minimal level of support yet others may need a great deal of support to successfully navigate a new phase of life.

As the mom (now legal guardian) of an adult daughter diagnosed with autism and an intellectual disability, transitions are complicated and her personal transitions often affect our family. She is unable to comprehend abstract concepts and her communication skills are limited. For her, times of transition tend to be filled with anxiety and confusion. It requires our active support which comes in the form of developing a solid plan to help the transition to go as smoothly as possible both practically and emotionally. It is important to recognize that transitions are not always related to the process of the transition itself, but about that fact that we are not always able to get our daughter's input when it is a complex situation that she cannot understand. We are aware that we have an enormous responsibility and therefore we need to consider these three issues as well: her safety, her health, and her happiness.

When making a transition, our goal is to determine the best way to smooth the path for her so that she can be successful. Over the years we have worked with excellent specialists. We talk through possible obstacles and then consider various options before we choose which path to take. It is often mentally and emotionally exhausting. We may develop a plan, but when we implement that plan, there is a great likelihood that obstacles arise that we had not considered and we then need to make modifications. It is a process.

There are times when a transition is not a "natural" one, but it affects us much more than it affects her. Her 30th birthday was one of those times. Though she became a legal adult at age 21, she was just out of school and that transition was more about moving to the adult system than it was about her chronologically becoming an adult. We felt like there was still plenty of time for us to teach her new skills and increase her independence. Then came her 30th birthday and it hit me hard. It felt like we were entering a new stage. I was feeling quite anxious so I had this idea that we should have a party. This initially increased my anxiety, however as we went through the process of planning, it felt right. We had support from amazing professionals and came up with a great plan that included a music therapist, a face painting artist, cake, and of course, some wonderful friends and their families. Seeing our gal celebrate and be celebrated was an amazing way to move into this new phase of her life with joy. It also brought home the concept of embracing transition—one that we will be trying to hold on to as we continue through many more transitions to come.

On a personal note, when Dr. Hart shared the premise of this book, I was excited and honored to be a small part of this project. The world of special needs (or special abilities, as I like to refer to it) is so complex. When we have the opportunity to learn more clearly what the hurdles may be and what can be effective, we can stretch our thinking in order to be supportive and helpful to individuals and their families. We should never be stuck with "because that's how we have always done it" kind of thinking. We need to grow with the research. This book will be a great catalyst for growth in the right direction.

Hartford, CT, USA   D. C.
September 2023

Acknowledgments

The initial research included in this book was conducted at the University of Auckland, New Zealand under the supervision of Honorary Associate Professor Mary Hill and Professor Janet Gaffney. International external examiners of the produced doctoral thesis (dissertation) were Professor Emerita Patricia O'Brien (Centre for Disability Studies, University of Sydney) and Professor Mary Morningstar (Professor of Education at Portland State University, Oregon). I would like to express my deepest appreciation to each of them, as well as Professor Audrey Trainor, for supporting the development of this project and myself as an academic. Furthermore, I am indebted to each of the young adult cases and their support networks for inviting me to capture their transition experiences. Appreciation is extended to the American Voices Project for access to their dataset and technical support. I'd like to recognize and thank the parent advocates who shared their valuable insights in the forward of the book. Thanks are also extended for support from the University of Hartford. To the Women's Advancement Initiative for research assistance funded through the Dorothy Goodwin Scholarship program. To the College of Education, Nursing, and Health Professions for funding and professional support, as well as to my supportive colleagues. Grateful acknowledgment to the editorial team at Palgrave Macmillan for their seamless cooperation in the publishing process, as well as the anonymous reviewers for their productive feedback. Lastly, my love and gratitude to my family. In particular, my father, the original Dr. Hart, for his red pen edits and guidance throughout the publication process. To Mark, Estelle, Graydon, Lux dog, and my family on both hemispheres, without your nurturing encouragement (and sense of adventure), this book would not have been possible.

CONTENTS

About the Author

Sarah M. Hart (PhD in Education) is Associate Professor of Special Education in the College of Education, Nursing, and Health Professions at the University of Hartford in Connecticut, USA. With a doctoral degree from the University of Auckland, New Zealand, she has lived, worked, studied, and taught in both countries. Her research is in the same area as her former teaching, post-school transitions for young adults with significant disabilities. She is now a teacher educator supporting those who work in these same fields. Her academic scholarship has been presented and published internationally, with specializations in equity in special education transition, disability studies and inclusion of individuals with significant disability, participatory and qualitative research methods, and social justice framed by capability approach.

LIST OF FIGURES

CHAPTER 1

Introduction

Abstract This chapter describes key terms vital to the central theme of dignity in post-school transition for young adults with significant disabilities. Dignity is defined within the capability approach framework and used to encompass the complexity of various transition domains and support systems. The intersectionality of disability and capability is examined. The author's positionality as a transition teacher and researcher adds depth to the discussion, acknowledging tensions within educational settings and personal experiences.

Keywords Active citizenship • Positionality • Post-school transition • Vulnerability

Imagine someone who uses a wheelchair for mobility. In an ideal situation, this person has individualized adaptive equipment, access to health and therapeutic care, and sufficient mobility routines. Their use of a wheelchair is not inherently problematic. Until one day this wheelchair-using individual comes to a building and there is no ramp to navigate past the front stairs. Or maybe the building has been entered, and the elevator is broken thus leaving the desired floor inaccessible. The challenges faced by this person are not within them or their adaptive equipment; but rather with the building itself. Now extend this metaphor further. Replace entry into a single building with the challenge of accessing one's entire community. Furthermore, replace wheelchair use with severe and complex needs. Because significant disability is far more complex than the use of a wheelchair, the issue of denied access extends well beyond inadequate physical accommodations. Historical segregation, stereotypes, and marginalization throughout most of the twentieth century have barred social access and meaningful community engagement (Albrecht, 1973). It is within this context that young adults with significant disabilities embark on their post-school life, a process often referred to in the education field simply as transition.

Key Terms

The key term dignity used in the book title signals the central commitment of this work. Defined through the capability approach (Nussbaum, 2000; Sen, 1999), dignity is the interaction between an individual's freedom to choose from a diverse capability set of opportunities, and the societal contexts whereby such freedoms eventuate in meaningful outcomes. This and other important terms related to transition policy, practice, and self-determination are defined here, and serve to provide a structure and rationale for the necessity of this work.

Transition Simply defined, a successful post-school transition from school involves that "the day after graduation should look no different than the day before for the individual exiting the school system" (Certo et al., 2008, p. 89). Yet the complexity of that seemingly simple task cuts across multiple domains (e.g., academic, vocational, interpersonal relationships, health), contexts (e.g., classrooms, workplaces, residential homes), time points (e.g., in-school and post-school), and support systems (e.g., schools, adult agencies, families, community supports; Carter et al., 2014). For students with and without disabilities, transition involves taking on new roles and adapting or changing existing roles (Osgood et al., 2005). Transition is more than an administrative procedure, biological life stage, or public policy issue. It implies a change in status, both in how we see ourselves and how others perceive us.

Transition can be marked by ending school, as well as by the beginning of "active citizenship" (Smith, 2013, p. 415) that emphasizes community engagement, individual autonomy, self-determination, and the right to participate in social and economic life. Note that the term citizenship is used to denote the goings on and engagement of people who collectively live in a place, not to prioritize the status of being from, or having an allegiance to, a particular country. The emphasis here is on the active nature of citizenship. A feeling of being included in the membership in one's community. Community participation, then, is not only a goal of post-school transition. It is also a "process by which other goals are achieved" (Emerson, 1985, cited in Myers et al., 1998, p. 390).

Research literature on post-school transition for students with disabilities is vast. One consistent concern is the many barriers and issues faced by young adults with disabilities (McCoy et al., 2020). Young people around the world experience disparities in the areas of employment, post-secondary education, and independent living, just to name a few. For example, when youth with and without disabilities are compared, those with disabilities who received a bachelor's degree were three times less likely to be employed (Mazzotti et al., 2021). Growing waiting lists for entry into support services add further strain to the situation, as do other influences such as poverty, culture, and marginalization (Trainor et al., 2020). When considered by such outcomes, youth with disabilities have restricted opportunities to fully participate in post-school, community life to the same degree as their non-disabled peers.

To address these concerns, educators support their students' planning and preparation for exiting secondary education, or high school, toward the next stage in young adulthood. This might include a two- or four-year college or technical training school, the workforce, a community-based or individualized program, or other options. Collaborative post-school planning is legally mandated for students with significant disabilities. In the teen years, plans are developed to understand and execute individual goals and desires of students to increase the likelihood of receiving appropriate occupational, social, and environmental supports. Yet, the challenge is to ensure that the hopes, goals, and perspective of the young adults at the center of transition is understood and actioned within these complex support systems (Hetherington et al., 2010).

Capability and Disability The target population of this research focuses on individuals with the highest 1% of most severe, profound, and multiple disabilities. To illustrate, one young adult case in this book has significant intellectual and developmental disabilities, coupled with severe autism, non-verbal communication, vision impairment, and unpredictable behaviors. During school, such students typically receive support for their communication and positive behavior through functional curriculums (highly modified to learn practical life skills) and community-based programs (shifting the academic learning space into the community that students will be graduating into). While these descriptions may pinpoint clarification, disability is far more than an individual's condition. Disability is socially and culturally constructed, and therefore disability terminology is contentious, varied, and intersectional.

Severe and complex needs have diverse and multidimensional impacts on quality of life. A further way to understand disability is in the interactions between the individual and their social contexts (Mitra, 2006). Capability approach considers what individuals can do, rather than what they cannot. It inclusively situates their contributions within social contexts. The capability approach can also be used to consider transition through the development and interaction of freedom and dignity. Essentially, as a matter of social justice.

Aotearoa New Zealand (ANZ) and the United States (USA) Through the lived experiences of youth in transition on two opposite sides of the globe, fresh understandings emerge about the topic of post-school transition. Researched before and during pandemic times, the central research question asks how the perspectives of individuals with significant disability can impact a transition with dignity? Answers to this question may be of interest to a wide scope of potential audiences including: parents, families, caregivers; teachers; teacher support personnel and administrators; social welfare services; transition support services and community service personnel; policy makers; social justice and disability advocates. While audiences from ANZ and USA may be particularly interested, the stories and experiences shared in this book are aimed to be accessible to those in the wider international community. In particular, themes of disability, inclusion, and human rights will hold high relevance to all.

Author Positionality My personal experiences as a transition teacher have prompted this research. I have worked as a certified transition teacher for over ten years in both ANZ and USA. The emphasis of my teaching was focused on community. I attempted to transform the school classroom into the very community students would enter after they left school. This was achieved through transition-aged students learning in community spaces (e.g., office blocks, public spaces such as libraries) instead of traditional classrooms, and utilizing community resources (e.g., public transportation, local sports clubs or gyms) instead of using school-based resources. I considered transition to be "successful" when the goals outlined in students' transition plans were achieved. I was concerned with outcomes. I wanted to know the students would end up "somewhere" after they finished school.

Despite the community-based aspects of transition, my career was predominantly based in special schools and segregated educational settings. By their very existence, these separate environments create a problematic tension of "institutionalized ableism" and the inherent need for segregation (Mutua & Smith, 2006, p. 129). Special educators and segregated educational environments reinforce a perceived need for parallel education systems due to a presumption of inherent difficulties of the students therein. Yet, these educational settings and systems still very much exist, and are sometimes a desirable option for students, their caregivers, and families. Applying logic from the capability approach (which will be further unpacked throughout the book), the choice to attend a segregated special school is not inherently problematic, unless the circumstances around that student's attendance were due to restrictions, such as no other educational options being offered or available.

As I am now a researcher and teacher-educator, I acknowledge these tensions. Through my background, I have access to experiences that make me an insider to a social world that few know much about. My educational experiences directly inform my current work as a teacher educator focused on inspiring a new generation of teachers to foster and further the development of schools that are inclusive, vibrant spaces, and school communities that thrive.

Lastly, I acknowledge that while conducting the research depicted in this book, I wore a metaphoric research armor that those participating in the research, either through fieldwork or interview, did not. Post-school transition is a tumultuous time. Oftentimes those closest to this critical life stage have the most emotionally complicated experiences. While I consider myself an emic insider to research in this field, I am also a relative outsider to the personal impact and influence on the individual outcomes of the transitions portrayed in this research. This is to say, this is not an intervention study where the outcomes of the observed transitions aimed to be changed. Instead, I hope that everyone reading this book connects with certain aspects of the depicted transition experiences, and finds ways to promote dignified changes within their own circumstances.

Chapter Summaries At first reading, the title *Transition with Dignity* may have suggested that transition experiences depicted within this book will solely represent positive and successful outcomes for individuals with disabilities. As a forewarning, note that this will not be the case. Life experiences are rarely so unequivocally straightforward, and the young adult cases in ANZ and USA were no exception. The term dignity directly signals the theoretical commitment of this work, yet it is not intended to refute the reality of disability experiences. The title has an aspirational purpose that will be discussed throughout each chapter, which are summarized as follows.

Chapter 2 delivers more depth into the topic of leaving school during the critical life stage of young adulthood. International contexts of Aotearoa New Zealand (ANZ) and United States (USA) will be described and then become the setting to define main concepts such as post-school transition and significant disability. The overall consideration will be the mechanisms that make for socially just and inclusive realities for those with significant disabilities.

Chapter 3 provides an in-depth examination of the capability framing of social justice, and describes its impacts on the research. Capability approach will also be applied to understand disability, post-school transition, as well as a method of international comparison. A novel way to examine individuals' exit from school to adult life is by defining transition as the way it expands an individual's capabilities.

Chapter 4 describes the methods of research inquiry. Qualitative data collection procedures portray a range of innovations used to facilitate the inclusion of individuals with significant disabilities in the research. In ANZ, classic ethnographic techniques were adapted to align with the communication preferences of those with disabilities to facilitate their agentic participation. In USA, data came from a secondary analysis of the American Voices Project qualitative dataset. Conducted through a joint initiative of Stanford and Princeton Universities, a nationally representative sample of interviews were collected during the pandemic lockdown. Findings are therefore uniquely applicable to current times of change. Capability and artifact analysis, as well as the process of member checks for credibility, will also be described. Steps to be inclusive in research can parallel community inclusion efforts.

Chapter 5 is the central heart of this book; case narrative portraits that are vividly described. Each narrative depicts lived transition experiences that portray the realities of leaving school for young adults with significant disabilities in both countries of ANZ and USA. A transition anchor tangibly joins the narratives together in an accessible manner.

Chapter 6 will begin by ascribing a metaphoric symbol of capability to each narrative. Reframed to focus on possibilities over problems, key themes of the dignity of risk and opportunity will be described. Together these themes culminate in understanding a transition with dignity.

Chapter 7 summarizes the central themes. Implications of the findings point to exciting opportunities to promote change.

"If a society is able to think through and successfully confront issues of disability, doing so will make it more compassionate, more secure in its sense of community, and more understanding both of human vulnerability and dependence and of human nature and potential" (Wolff, 2009, p. 148).

References

Albrecht, G. L. (1973). Socialization in the rehabilitation process. *Health Services Research, 8*(1), 67.

Carter, E. W., Brock, M. E., & Trainor, A. A. (2014). Transition assessment and planning for youth with severe intellectual and developmental disabilities. *The Journal of Special Education, 47*(4), 245–255. https://doi.org/10.1177/0022466912456241

Certo, N. J., Luecking, R. G., Murphy, S., Brown, L., Courey, S., & Belanger, D. (2008). Seamless transition and long-term support for individuals with severe intellectual disabilities. *Research and Practice for Persons with Severe Disabilities, 33*(3), 85–95. https://doi.org/10.2511/rpsd.33.3.85

Hetherington, S. A., Durant-Jones, L., Johnson, K., Nolan, K., Smith, E., Taylor-Brown, S., & Tuttle, J. (2010). The lived experiences of adolescents with disabilities and their parents in transition planning. *Focus on Autism and Other Developmental Disabilities, 25*(3), 163–172. https://doi.org/10.1177/1088357610373760

Mazzotti, V. L., Rowe, D. A., Kwiatek, S., Voggt, A., Chang, W.-H., Fowler, C. H., Poppen, M., Sinclair, J., & Test, D. W. (2021). Secondary transition predictors of postschool success: An update to the research base. *Career Development and Transition for Exceptional Individuals, 44*(1), 47–64. https://doi.org/10.1177/2165143420959793

McCoy, S., Shevlin, M., & Rose, R. (2020). Secondary school transition for students with special educational needs in Ireland. *European Journal of Special Needs Education, 35*(2), 154–170. https://doi.org/10.1080/08856257.2019.1628338

Mitra, S. (2006). The capability approach and disability. *Journal of Disability Policy Studies, 16*(4), 236–247. https://doi.org/10.1177/10442073060160040501

Mutua, K., & Smith, R. M. (2006). Disrupting normalcy and the practical concerns of classroom teachers. In S. Danforth & S. L. Gabel (Eds.), *Vital questions facing disability studies in education* (1st ed., pp. 121–132). Lang.

Myers, F., Ager, A., Kerr, P., & Myles, S. (1998). Outside looking in? Studies of the community integration of people with learning disabilities. *Disability and Society, 13*(3), 389–413. https://doi.org/10.1080/09687599826704

Nussbaum, M. C. (2000). *Women and human development: The capabilities approach.* Cambridge University Press.

Osgood, W., Foster, E. M., Flanagan, C., & Ruth, G. R. (2005). *On your own without a net: The transition to adulthood for vulnerable populations.* University of Chicago Press.

Sen, A. (1999). *Development as freedom.* Oxford University Press.

Smith, S. R. (2013). Citizenship and disability: Incommensurable lives and wellbeing. *Critical Review of International Social and Political Philosophy, 16*(3), 403–420. https://doi.org/10.1080/13698230.2013.795708

Trainor, A. A., Carter, E. W., Karpur, A., Martin, J. E., Mazzotti, V. L., Morningstar, M. E., & Rojewski, J. W. (2020). A framework for research in transition: Identifying important areas and intersections for future study. *Career Development and Transition for Exceptional Individuals, 43*(1), 5–17. https://doi.org/10.1177/21651434198645

Wolff, J. (2009). Cognitive disability in a society of equals. *Metaphilosophy, 40*(3-4), 402–415. https://doi.org/10.1111/j.1467-9973.2009.01598.x

CHAPTER 2

International Contexts of School Leaving

Abstract In this chapter, an overview of public education systems in Aotearoa New Zealand and the USA focuses on disability-related services during the culminating school years. Transition functions within each country are then described through available post-school options and services that promote the successful post-school lives of those with disabilities. Lastly, the meaning and nature of disability is examined for both settings, including practical implications for those living and supporting transition.

Keywords Aotearoa New Zealand (ANZ) • Models of disability • Inclusion • Quality of life domains • Research literature • United States of America (USA)

"Transition from adolescence to adulthood is a period of time pregnant with paradoxes" (Trainor, 2017, p. 1). Often referred to through the metaphor of a bridge, post-school transition is a liminal developmental stage crossing both in-school and post-school settings. Too commonly, however, themetaphor associated with transition is "falling off a cliff" (Davies & Beam ish, 2009, p. 249). Despite years of transition research, post-school outcomes remain unacceptably poor in areas such as enrollment into post-secondary education, employment rates, and inclusion in community-based activities (Trainor et al., 2020). The severity of the problem increases with the severity or complexity of one's disability.

Aotearoa New Zealand (ANZ)

Aotearoa New Zealand (indigenous Māori terms and country name will be used unless describing a specific document or agency) is in the South Pacific. The physical country is part of the wider region known as Australasia and Oceania, not on the continent of Australia. The country's largest inhabited islands are Te Ika-a-Māui North Island, and Te Waipounamu South Island, with fewer people living on smaller islands around the country.

ANZ is one of the last major landmasses settled by humans, first inhabited by Eastern Polynesians between 1250 and 1300. Those early settlers developed a distinct culture now known as Māori. The first European known to reach ANZ was a Dutch explorer, Abel Tasman, in 1642, then again in 1769 when British explorer, Captain James Cook, mapped almost the entire coastline. The Treaty of Waitangi was signed between Māori chiefs and the British Crown on 6 February 1840, and on 1 July 1841 ANZ became a separate British colony. The year 1948 was the first time those living in the country became New Zealand citizens, before then they had been British citizens. Full legal independence was gained when Parliament passed the Constitution Act in 1986 (Belich, 2001).

The country operates under a parliamentary system with executive power held by a Cabinet. The Cabinet is led by the Prime Minister. ANZ is notable for being the first country in the world to give women the right to vote in 1893 and has been identified as one of the world's most stable, transparent, and least corrupt nations (Transparency International, 2022).

Before the establishment of a state education system in 1877, education in ANZ was held in houses of learning where traditional Māori knowledge was shared. From 1816, Missionaries developed provincial schools to teach Māori to read and develop their oral language into written form. Now, the Organisation for Economic Co-operation and Development ranked ANZ within the world's top 20 nations for the quality of public schools (OECD, 2022). Early childhood education operates from birth to school entry age. It is not compulsory, but around 95% of children attend some form of early childhood education service that operates from a national curriculum known as Te Whāriki (Ministry of Education, 2023).

Between ages 3 and 5, a child is subsidized to attend 20 hours of early childhood education for free. Primary education begins on a child's fifth birthday and is compulsory from ages 6 to 16. The education system is made up of 13-year levels, with primary education starting at Year 1 and going to Year 8 (approximately ages 5–12), and secondary going from Year 9 to Year 13 (approximately ages 13–17). State schools are allocated funding from the Government on a per-student basis to support the operation of the school. Schools receive funding based on a school's socioeconomic decile rating on a scale of 1 (lowest) to 10 (highest). Approximately 10% of schools are in each decile ranking. The lower the decile ranking, the more funding a school receives. All schools also receive a Special Education Grant issued as part of their general operations to be used autonomously to best meet the needs of their students. The Ministry of Education is the lead advisor to the Government on education.

Education is pivotal for achieving the aim of a fully inclusive society. The country signed the United Nations Convention on the Rights of Persons with Disabilities (UNCRPD) in 2006 and ratified to extend protocols in 2008. Through 50 articles and amendments, leadership, coordination, and accountability for implementation ensures to promote and protect the full and equal enjoyment of all human rights, fundamental freedoms, and dignity of persons with disabilities. The UNCRPD is the central focus for the New Zealand Disability Strategy, Outcomes Framework, and Disability Action Plan. Education is one of eight interconnected outcomes of the Disability Action Plan (Office of Disability Issues, 2023).

For students with more significant special needs, an application is made for external assessment to gain access to Ongoing Resourcing Scheme (ORS) funding. ORS funding is individually targeted to support students with the highest 3% of significant needs, and there are two levels, high and very high. Each denote the significance of ongoing or extreme needs in the areas of: learning, hearing, vision, physical disability, and/or language use and social communication. Access to ORS funding provides support for individual students including specialists, additional teaching supports (e.g., paraprofessional teachers), and consumable resources. Students receiving ORS funding also have a collaboratively created Individualized Education Plan (IEP). Notably, this funding mechanism does not rely on diagnosis, nor is a disability classification, or label, to receive services (Gaffney et al., 2017).

In 2018, a comprehensive rollout of the Enabling Good Lives initiative transformed disability support systems. This has been further bolstered by the creation of Whaikaha, a new Ministry of Disabled People. The primary focus is to break down the previously fragmented social welfare system across the various ministries involved in the lives of people with disabilities. For example, in the case of transition, to forge partnerships that wrap a range of supports around an individual's personal needs (Whaikaha, 2023).

United States of America (USA)

While operating on the assumption that most will have a foundational understanding of the workings of USA, there is one crucial influence on the country's functional practices, including education, that is worth further explanation. USA is a federal republic composed of 50 states, plus additional territories, which essentially forms a division of power between federal and state governments. Importantly, each state has a sovereign government with certain powers to act autonomously from the federal government. Pertinent impacts of this governmental structure on the education sector include funding and organizational structures of public schools, implementation of federal mandates, age ranges of school students, as well as teacher preparation and certification (The White House, 2023).

The foundation of special education in America is based on the civil rights established in the landmark case of Brown vs. the Board of Education. Separate is not equal. Therefore, students with disabilities should have access to attend the same schools in the same classrooms as their peers without disabilities. Students observed or suspected of having a disability can be referred by teachers, parents, and others for a comprehensive assessment to determine educational supports (Aron & Loprest, 2012). Eligibility criteria for a specific disability category (of which there are 13) can be set by each state so long as a nondiscriminatory evaluation is ensured. The Individuals with Disabilities Education Act (IDEA), first passed in 1975, is the federal law that ensures the public education of all students with disabilities. IDEA safeguards students' access to a Free and Appropriate Public Education (FAPE) in the Least Restrictive Environment (LRE). An Individualized Education Program (IEP) is collaboratively created and aligned to the individual services, interventions, and curricular needs of each student.

With specific attention to transition, IDEA requires that students from age 16 (or younger depending on the state) outline the specific steps they will take to develop functional skills for work and community life that are based on student's strengths, preferences, and interests. Within applicable parts of the IEP, a statement of transition service needs must be articulated. For example, pre-requisite courses needed to enroll in post-secondary education should be arranged. Transition planning also involves preparation for when a young person reaches the age of majority, with plans for who will hold the rights to decision-making and legal implications (Office of Special Education and Rehabilitative Services, 2020).

DESCRIPTION OF POST-SCHOOL TRANSITION

Students experience many transitions during their school years, for instance, the transition from early childhood education into primary or elementary school. In this section, post-school transition is considered in a few ways. First, the IDEA definition of transition in USA is provided. Next key domains involved in transition are examined in both settings of ANZ and USA. Lastly, contemporary international empirical scholarship is reviewed.

In Section 300.43 of the IDEA, the following definition of transition is provided that directly impacts much of the transition-related education services in USA to this day.

Transition services means a coordinated set of activities for a child with a disability that

(1) is designed to be within a results-oriented process, that is focused on improving the academic and functional achievement of the child with a disability to facilitate the child's movement from school to post-school activities, including postsecondary education, vocational education, integrated employment (including supported employment), continuing and adult education, adult services, independent living, or community participation;

(2) is based on the individual child's needs, taking into account the child's strengths, preferences, and interests; and includes:

(i) instruction;
(ii) related services;
(iii) community experiences;

    (iv) the development of employment and other post-school adult living objectives; and

    (v) if appropriate, acquisition of daily living skills and provision of a functional vocational evaluation.

Transition services for children with disabilities may be special education, if provided as specially designed instruction, or a related service, if required to assist a child with a disability to benefit from special education (Office of Special Education and Rehabilitative Services, 2020).

Six sections of IDEA cover important transition topics such as when and how to include transition goals and objectives in the IEP; transition services; IEP team composition; transfer of rights at age of majority; and requirements for exiting high school programs. Yet, policy, especially the policies of one particular country, don't sufficiently portray the complexity of transition. To provide a context and comparison of transition in both ANZ and USA, key quality of life domains of life, settings, supports, and services are here considered.

Life and settings The domains of life and setting share similarities between the two countries of ANZ and USA. While an exit from compulsory schooling can be seen as a momentous life achievement for some, for others, such as individuals with severe and complex needs, the exit from school is another instance of aging out (Osgood et al., 2005). Aging out has multiple implications.

In transition, aging out signals students who are not necessarily graduating school because of merit, completion of standards, or even due to days of attendance. These young adults are leaving school for no reason or marker other than their age. Transition programs in both ANZ and USA run until approximately age 21 (though age varies slightly by the state in USA). The age of school leaving impacts students with disabilities because transition becomes a time when they can continue to access secondary, high school past the age of their non-disabled peers who typically complete school around age 18. Thus, in-school settings become increasingly outgrown and inappropriate as common transition settings prioritize community integration for leisure, employment, or day programs. For instance, transition classes are sometimes held on college or university campuses, or in community halls or spaces like a town library.

In both countries, transition also involves shifting to adult-oriented services. For instance, leaving pediatric medical practices to receive care from a general medical practitioner. Another more complicated example is the consideration of enduring guardianship, as peers without disabilities typically manage their own guardianship upon reaching the age of majority at 18. Such decisions hold implications for civic participation, such as voting rights, as well as accountability matters, such as adult criminal justice systems.

Supports Transition practices begin to diverge between ANZ and USA when considered through the domain of transition supports. Both countries rely heavily on what is known in the field as interagency collaboration, support providers who operate from both in and outside of the school as they create and implement transition plans. With the student at the center, members of interagency support teams typically include parents or caregivers and family, teachers, specialized services, and community service providers. One distinction between the countries is the role of transition coordinators, practitioners who work with students with disabilities to support their post-school goals (Scheef & Mahfouz, 2020). Whereas special education teachers focus on the academic and social needs of their students, a transition coordinator has a role outside of supporting academic skills, and may even continue their services after the completion of school. In ANZ the transition coordinator role is available in the final year of school. Transition students with disability and their families can broker a transition coordinator for one full year of transition supports that typically bridge the in-school to post-school changeover. It is more common in USA, however, that school administration and special educators manage transition supports (Scheef & Mahfouz, 2020). In USA, transition planning will begin approximately five years before school leaving, but school-based supports conclude when school does.

Despite the procedures and structure, interagency collaboration teams are universally challenging to manage in practice (Plotner et al., 2020). Consequences of ineffective collaborations are location-specific, however. In ANZ, teachers are siloed and therefore primarily distant or sometimes completely absent from the planning and preparation of their students' transitions (Hart et al., 2015). This is due, in part, to the shift in the priority for community support personnel who are primarily responsible for care after the young adult completes school. It may also be an unintended consequence of the transition coordinator role that potentially sidelines the necessity for teachers' participation. In USA, since teachers and school administration primarily lead transition, they often centralize school personnel in the planning (Plotner et al., 2020). While relevant community service providers legally need to be invited to collaborate, Plotner and colleagues found that teachers did not fully understand the roles of certain outside agencies. This led to breakdowns in interagency collaboration, which inhibited communication and slowed productivity.

Services Another subtle distinction between the two countries is the transition service support structures. In ANZ, transition signals the end of funding from the Ministry of Education, and marks an increase in funding sourced from the Ministries of Health and Social Development. This shift is notable, not only because it is the prerequisite for a reassessment of functional care needs, but also because the funding between ministries varies greatly. For instance, the Ministry of Health receives far more funding than the Ministry of Social Development.

Transition in USA involves legal shifts. Student protections under the IDEA are no longer relevant once a young adult completes school. Legal protections are then covered by the Americans with Disabilities (ADA). ADA offers more global protections such as non-discrimination in areas such as the workplace, community building codes, and public transportation. Akin to the discrepancy in ministry funding in ANZ, the challenge is that ADA does not receive the same financial support as IDEA. Therefore, transitioning students who exit services under IDEA experience a significant decrease in financial support under ADA. For example, a student accustomed to modified curriculum with vast in-school accommodations can only expect basic academic supports (e.g., extended time on tests, alternative testing locations) should they choose to enroll in post-secondary education.

Empirical research literature Another way to situate the current context of post-school transition is through academic literature. Before presenting the reviewed literature two acknowledgements are that: (1) A comprehensive historical review of transition scholarship is not provided. The emphasis, rather, is to provide a succinct contemporary snapshot of new directions in transition research. For a broad, historical review of seminal work in the field, please see scholars such as Shogren and Wehmeyer (2020); Sitlington et al. (2010); or Trainor (2017). (2) Compiling international literature was the aim. However, the knowledge base is admittedly skewed toward USA since the majority of academic journals, and thus transition literature, originate from there.

For over 40 years, multiple waves of nationally representative large-scale studies have tracked the experiences of young adults in USA. Called the National Longitudinal Transition Study (NLTS, 1989; NLTS2, 2009), ten years of data following each cohort's conclusion from school has illustrated an overall pattern that when compared to non-disabled peers, youth with disabilities are less likely to have positive post-school experiences across a range of social, professional, and engagement markers. To address these concerns, specific in-school transition practices have been studied for their impact on post-school outcomes (Test et al., 2009). The NLTS articulated a list of positive practices or "predictors" such as: career technical education; inclusion in general education; self-care, goal-setting life skills instruction; paid employment/work experience; and self-determination skill instruction, to name a few (Newman et al., 2011). Over time, these outcome predictors have shifted, increased, and become more nuanced (Mazzotti et al., 2021). For example, having "psychological empowerment" defined as one's understanding and belief in a relationship between actions and outcomes, is now understood for the significant ways in which it impacts the longstanding practice of promoting students' self-determination (Mazzotti et al., 2021, p. 48).

Another emerging area of focus is on the intersectional identities of diverse young adults with disabilities (i.e., the interconnected nature of social categorizations such as race, class, gender, etc. as they apply to a given individual or group). By bringing diverse cultural backgrounds to the forefront of transition, issues such as exclusionary discipline procedures and access to healthcare have become important matters for consideration (Trainor et al., 2019). One strategy to incorporate intersectional identities is to implement culturally sustaining educational practices. Typically, culturally sustaining practices focus on the promotion of academic achievement through intentional school pedagogy that develops cultural competence (Paris, 2021). Culturally sustaining practices in transition can mirror these efforts through the invitation, involvement, and encouragement of cultural practices and aspects of home cultures throughout students' preparation to leave school.

Another recurrent point in the contemporary transition literature is interagency collaboration (a theme that has already been directly compared within ANZ and USA with divergent results). Collaborations between schools and vocational rehabilitation (or pre-employment preparation) agencies, however, are "uneven and fairly limited" (Carter et al., 2021, p. 161). Educators have been found to skew their views based on school level (i.e., middle versus high school) and community type (i.e., rural versus non-rural). In another study, students with milder, or less visible impacts of autism (formerly called Asperger's) were found less likely to transition to college after leaving school despite their academic abilities to do so (Alverson et al., 2019). Oftentimes these outcomes derive from decisions made after limited supports are provided in domains such as: motivation, disability awareness, family supports, coordinated transition planning, and associated post-school goals.

Brought together, recent literature on intersectional identity and interagency collaboration indicates that, unfortunately, "transition education is not a panacea for inequality" (Trainor, 2017, p. 124). While in-school practices can aim to improve post-school outcomes, they do not sufficiently address the hopes, dreams, and needs of today's youth. Transition is therefore more than simply procedural. It depends as much upon in-school procedures and systems as it does on the inclusivity of society itself. To reexamine transition in a new light requires firstly a fundamental reconsideration of the meaning and nature of disability itself.

DESCRIPTION OF DISABILITY

"For much of history, disability has been understood in negative terms as pathology, aberration, and something atypical" (Wehmeyer & Patton, 2017, p. 4). The already introduced UNCRPD and the World Health Organization have both made strides in challenging historical models for defining disability. A broadened concept of disability is to now consider the reciprocal interaction between the environment and a person's capacities.

The two countries of ANZ and USA define disability in distinct ways. In USA, the definition of disability is aligned through the assessment and diagnostic criteria of IDEA. To receive services, qualified professionals individually assess students who must fall within one of 13 pre-determined disability categories including labels such as Specific Learning Disability, Autism Spectrum, or Other Health Impairments. By contrast, ANZ distinguishes between disability and impairments:

Disability is not something individuals have. What individuals have are impairments. They may be physical, sensory, neurological, psychiatric, intellectual, or other impairments. Disability is the process which happens when one group of people create barriers by designing a world only for their way of living, taking no account of the impairments other people have. (Whaikaha, 2023)

Within these definitions, the two countries poignantly differentiate between two differing conceptual models of disability, the medical and social. Classification mechanisms in USA align with a medicalized model. Disability exists within an individual who requires sustained remediation and care provided by professionals who create individual treatment plans. Disability management under a medical model is aimed at a "cure," or as close to operational normalcy as possible. The emphasis is therefore on access to effective medical care, treatments, and therapy. ANZ's definition is illustrative of a social orientation of disability. People with individual impairments are disabled by society, whether by design, principles, or practices, more so than by their own bodies or differences (Shakespeare, 2018). Addressing systemic barriers is the way to improve conditions for those with disabilities.

The cultural shift from a medical to social conceptual orientation illustrates developments in the way that disability is defined and therefore addressed. Collectively, there is a movement away from a welfare orientation in favor of human rights. The interplay between individual impairments, systemic barriers, and far more constructs a complex and diverse scope of the lived experiences of disability. Simply said, "impairment and impact are socially brokered" (Hopper, 2007, p. 870). This idea will be further explored in the next chapter regarding the capability approach. For now, however, the broadened scope disability marks important implications for the novel ways of understanding.

Inclusive disability research We should not "know" for others. Yet, individuals with severe, profound, and multiple disabilities are far too often positioned as subjects *for* research or completely side-lined altogether (Seale et al., 2014). Inclusive disability research emphasizes active engagement, and dismantling of an all too common perception that the more significant the disability, the more barriers exist to participation in educational research (Taylor, 2018). Done well, inclusive research design can facilitate collaborations between those with and without disabilities and ensure personal agency throughout the process.

Used here as an umbrella term, inclusive research encapsulates a range of research epistemologies and frameworks that are not exclusively disability-specific, including participatory, action research, emancipatory, and collaborative co-research, to name a few. Collectively considered, these approaches typically focus on amplifying the perspectives of a historically marginalized population. Individuals with disabilities are therefore "experts by experience" (Bigby et al., 2014, p. 59) as well as the primary users of research findings. Practically speaking, inclusive design employs a wide variety of approaches that position individuals with disabilities to serve in advisory or collaborative roles, including initiating, designing, and leading research studies (Bigby et al., 2014). The research depicted within this book joins a steadily increasing knowledge base of inclusive disability scholarship that seeks to understand the issues that matter to individuals with disabilities and aims to directly apply understandings to the improvement of their lives and experiences.

Chapter Conclusion

The countries of ANZ and USA have unique histories and educational backgrounds. Some key distinctions include the way disability is defined, and whether or not a discrete disability label is required to receive services. Additionally, the rights that undergird both country's transition policies differ. Descriptions were provided about the moral principles or human rights of transition, as well as the laws that ensure the civil rights of individuals in transition.

When made a "medicalized" commodity, transition focuses on remediating what is lacking in the individual. When focused on a social model of disability, transition can address the barriers to an inclusive society. Yet, a lack of understanding exists of the implications of transition policies and practices on the lived experiences of transition. Thus, a need for inclusive research exists to examine school leaving for the ways that preparations and practices can promote a thriving, post-school life for all.

References

Alverson, C. Y., Lindstrom, L. E., & Hirano, K. A. (2019). High school to college: Transition experiences of young adults with autism. *Focus on Autism and Other Developmental Disabilities, 34*(1), 52–64. https://doi.org/10.1177/1088357615611880

Aron, L., & Loprest, P. (2012). Disability and the education system. *The Future of Children, 22*(1), 97–122. https://www.jstor.org/stable/41475648

Belich, J. (2001). *Paradise reforged: A history of the New Zealanders from 1880 to the Year 2000.* Penguin Books.

Bigby, C., Frawley, P., & Ramcharan, P. (2014). Conceptualizing inclusive research with people with intellectual disability. *Journal of Applied Research in Intellectual Disabilities, 27*, 3–12. https://doi.org/10.1111/jar.12083

Carter, E. W., Awsumb, J. M., Schutz, M. A., & McMillan, E. D. (2021). Preparing youth for the world of work: Educator perspectives on pre-employment transition services. *Career Development and Transition for Exceptional Individuals, 44*(3), 161–173. https://doi.org/10.1177/2165143420938663

Davies, M. D., & Beamish, W. (2009). Transitions from school for young adults with intellectual disability: Parental perspectives on "life as an adjustment". *Journal of Intellectual and Developmental Disability, 34*(3), 248–257. https://doi.org/10.1080/13668250903103676

Gaffney, J. S., Morton, M., & Hart, S. M. (2017). Aotearoa New Zealand. In J. Patton & M. Wehmeyer (Eds.), *Handbook of international special education* (Vol. 3). Santa Barbara, CA.

Hart, S. M., Hill, M. F., & Gaffney, J. S. (2015). Teachers absent: Impacts upon the transition of students with significant special needs. In D. Garbett & A. Ovens (Eds.), *Teaching for tomorrow today* (pp. 491–498). Edify.

Hopper, K. (2007). Rethinking social recovery in schizophrenia: What a capabilities approach might offer. *Social Science and Medicine, 65*(5), 868–879. https://doi.org/10.1016/j.socscimed.2007.04.012

Institute of Education Sciences, National Center for Special Education Research (1989). *National longitudinal transition study.* Author: Retrieved from: https://nces.ed.gov/pubsearch/pubsinfo.asp?pubid=NCEE20154014

Institute of Education Sciences, National Center for Special Education Research (2009). *National longitudinal transition study-2.* Author: Retrieved from: https://ies.ed.gov/ncser/projects/nlts2/

Mazzotti, V. L., Rowe, D. A., Kwiatek, S., Voggt, A., Chang, W.-H., Fowler, C. H., Poppen, M., Sinclair, J., & Test, D. W. (2021). Secondary transition predictors of postschool success: An update to the research base. *Career Development and Transition for Exceptional Individuals, 44*(1), 47–64. https://doi.org/10.1177/2165143420959793

Ministry of Education. (2023). *Education in New Zealand: Our education system.* Author. Retrieved from: https://www.education.govt.nz/our-work/our-role-and-our-people/education-in-nz/

Newman, L. A, Wagner, M., Knokey, A., Marder, C., Nagle, K., Shaver, D., Wei, X., Cameto, R., Contreras, E., Ferguson, K., Greenes, S., & Schwarting, M. (2011). *The post-high school outcomes of young adults with disabilities up to 8 years after high school. A report from the National Longitudinal Transition Study-2 (NLTS2) (NCSER 2011—3005).* U. S. Department of Education. https://files.eric.ed.gov/fulltext/ ED524044.pdf

Office for Disability Issues. (2023). *Disability action plan 2019 – 2023.* Retrieved from: https://www.odi.govt.nz/disability-action-plan-2/

Office of Special Education and Rehabilitative Services, United States Department of Education. (2020). *A transition guide: To postsecondary education and employment for students and youth with disabilities.* District of Columbia.

Organisation for Economic Co-operation and Development. (2022). *Education at a glance: Education GPS.* Paris. Retrieved from: https://www.oecd.org/education/education-at-a-glance/

Osgood, W., Foster, E. M., Flanagan, C., & Ruth, G. R. (2005). *On your own without a net: The transition to adulthood for vulnerable populations.* University of Chicago Press.

Paris, D. (2021). Culturally sustaining pedagogies and our futures. *The Educational Forum, 85*(4), 364–376. https://doi.org/10.1080/00131725.2021.1957634

Plotner, A. J., Mazzotti, V. L., Rose, C. A., & Teasley, K. (2020). Perceptions of interagency collaboration: Relationships between secondary transition roles, communication, and collaboration. *Remedial and Special Education, 41*(1), 28–39. https://doi.org/10.1177/0741932518778029

Scheef, A., & Mahfouz, J. (2020). Supporting the post-school goals of youth with disabilities through use of a transition coordinator. *Research in Educational Administration and Leadership, 5*(1), 43–69. https://doi.org/10.30828/real/2020.1.2

Seale, J., Nind, M., & Parsons, S. (2014). Inclusive research in education: Contributions to method and debate. *International Journal of Research and Method in Education, 37*(4), 347–356. https://doi.org/10.1080/1743727X.2014.935272

Shakespeare, T. (2018). *Disability: The basics.* Routledge.

Shogren, K. A., & Wehmeyer, M. L. (2020). *Handbook of adolescent transition education for youth with disabilities* (2nd ed.). Routledge.

Sitlington, P. L., Neubert, D. A., & Clark, G. M. (2010). *Transition education and services for students with disabilities* (5th ed.). Pearson.

Taylor, A. (2018). Knowledge citizens? Intellectual disability and the production of social meanings within educational research. *Harvard Educational Review, 88*(1), 1–25. https://doi.org/10.17763/1943-5045-88.1.1

Test, D. W., Mazzotti, V. L., Mustian, A. L., Fowler, C. H., Kortering, L. J., & Kohler, P. H. (2009). Evidence based secondary transition predictors for improving postschool outcomes for students with disabilities. *Career Development for Exceptional Individuals, 32*, 160–181. https://doi.org/10.1177/0885728809346960

The White House. (2023). *Our Government*. District of Columbia. Retrieved from: https://www.whitehouse.gov/about-the-white-house/our-government/.

Trainor, A. A. (2017). *Transition by design: Improving equity and outcomes for adolescents with disabilities*. Teachers College Press.

Trainor, A. A., Newman, L., Garcia, E., Woodley, H. H., Traxler, R. E., & Deschene, D. N. (2019). Postsecondary education-focused transition planning experiences of English learners with disabilities. *Career Development and Transition for Exceptional Individuals, 42*(1), 43–55. https://doi.org/10.1177/2165143418811830

Trainor, A. A., Carter, E. W., Karpur, A., Martin, J. E., Mazzotti, V. L., Morningstar, M. E., & Rojewski, J. W. (2020). A framework for research in transition: Identifying important areas and intersections for future study. *Career Development and Transition for Exceptional Individuals, 43*(1), 5–17. https://doi.org/10.1177/21651434198645

Transparency International. (2022). *Corruption perceptions index*. Berlin. Retrieved from: https://www.transparency.org/en/cpi/2022

Wehmeyer, M., & Patton, J. (2017). *Handbook of international special education*. Praeger.

Whaikaha, Ministry of Disabled People. (2023). *Who we are*. Wellington. Retrieved from: https://www.whaikaha.govt.nz/about-us/who-we-are/

CHAPTER 3

Capability

Abstract In this chapter, the capability approach is introduced through the work of Amartya Sen and Martha Nussbaum. Capability will be described as a measure of international human development through its conceptualization, history, and prior research. From these understandings, capability forms the theoretical underpinning to this work by giving priority to the conditions that precede post-school transition regardless of how "successful" these outcomes are determined to be.

Keywords Capability approach • Freedom • Functionings • Opportunity

The prior chapter illustrated that active citizenship of individuals with significant disabilities following their exit from school depends as much upon in-school systematic procedures as it does the inclusivity of society itself. While supporting individual transition outcomes (e.g., employment rates, post-secondary education completion) are important, the promotion and enhancement of an inclusive society can be an integral to address the transition challenges faced by those with disabilities. In both ANZ and USA, however, more understanding is needed on the mechanisms that contribute to socially just and inclusive realities. Such shifts can directly impact the way disability is defined, and thereby the models used to frame our actions.

THEORETICAL FRAMEWORK

The capability approach was developed by Amartya Sen, who won the Nobel Prize in Economic Sciences in 1989 for creating this intentionally under-specified, normative framework for welfare economics. The approach focuses on the freedom to choose between individual capabilities to establish a life of personal value. As a measure of economic development, Sen took issue with aggregate measures of a country's growth such as wealth classifications like Gross Domestic Product (GDP). While a country's GDP may be a sign that the economy is doing well, Sen noted this does not inherently translate to positive experiences for people living there. In the capability approach, the unit of concern is every human being in their own right. "Human beings are not merely a means of production, but also the end of the exercise" (Sen, 1999, p. 296).

Central distinctions of capability approach are: (a) capability, what a person can do, be, and finds personally meaningful; (b) freedom, a person's actual freedoms to select from personally relevant opportunities that form an individual's capability set; and (c) functionings, the beings and doings of a person's life from the realization of their choices (Sen, 1999, p.6). Development, according to Sen, focuses on more than on individual outcomes, but rather on opportunities to achieve personal capabilities. To illustrate, Sen used a simple, yet poignant distinction between a starving person and a fasting person. Both people have the same shared outcome of hunger but for two very different reasons. The starving individual experiences hunger because of restricted access and opportunity to acquire nutrients and food, whereas the fasting person chooses to be hungry.

This example of hunger illustrates that interventions are insufficient when they are focused solely on outcomes such as goods, services, and resources. While these may "enable functioning" (Sen, 1999, p. 296) to use capability terminology, individual access may not be desired nor guaranteed. Additionally, it cannot be assumed that individuals will have the freedom to manage these means in alignment with their personal interests. Through the lens of capability, crucial considerations of genuine access need to be considered across a range of matters, such as environmental changes, like climate, physical surroundings, and infrastructure (all matters of increasing global concern). Social considerations are also critical, such as norms, public policies, or laws and mandates. To summarize Sen's approach, the focus is on each person's access, freedom, and choice within their own capability set, regardless of age, gender, ability, etc. Additionally, capabilities should not be contrived by other people's influence, whether that pertains to, for example, one spouse overseeing decisions for another, or caregivers making choices on behalf of those with disabilities without their consultation.

Philosopher and legal scholar, Martha Nussbaum worked from the same basic tenets of capability as Sen but emphasized the distribution of wealth, opportunities, and privileges within a society: all notions of social justice. Nussbaum used ten capabilities to universalize fundamental human rights and principles that she argued allowed for the greatest good for all human beings. This list is the same for everyone, those with and without disabilities alike. A threshold level of each listed capability is needed to establish a life of dignity. The ten central human capabilities are:

1. Life. Being able to live to the end of a human life of normal length; not dying prematurely, or before one's life is so reduced as to be not worth living.
2. Bodily health. Being able to have good health, including reproductive health; to be adequately nourished; to have adequate shelter.
3. Bodily integrity. Being able to move freely from place to place; to be secure against violent assault, including sexual assault and domestic violence; having opportunities for sexual satisfaction and for choice in matters of reproduction.
4. Senses, imagination, and thought. Being able to use the senses, to imagine, think, and reason—and to do these things in a "truly human" way, a way informed and cultivated by an adequate education, including, but by no means limited to, literacy and basic mathematical and scientific training. Being able to use imagination and thought in connection with experiencing and producing works and events of one's own choice, religious, literary, musical, and so forth. Being able to use one's mind in ways protected by guarantees of freedom of expression with respect to both political and artistic speech, and freedom of religious exercise. Being able to have pleasurable experiences and to avoid non-beneficial pain.
5. Emotions. Being able to have attachments to things and people outside ourselves; to love those who love and care for us, to grieve at their absence; in general, to love, to grieve, to experience longing, gratitude, and justified anger. Not having one's emotional development blighted by fear and anxiety. (Supporting this capa-

bility means supporting forms of human association that can be shown to be crucial in their development.)

6. Practical reason. Being able to form a conception of the good and to engage in critical reflection about the planning of one's life. (This entails protection for the liberty of conscience and religious observance.)

7. Affiliation. Being able to live with and toward others, to recognize and show concern for other humans, to engage in various forms of social interaction; to be able to imagine the situation of another. (Protecting this capability means protecting institutions that constitute and nourish such forms of affiliation, and also protecting the freedom of assembly and political speech). Having the social bases of self-respect and non-humiliation; being able to be treated as a dignified being whose worth is equal to that of others. This entails provisions of non-discrimination on the basis of race, sex, sexual orientation, ethnicity, caste, religion, national origin, and species.

8. Other species. Being able to live with concern for and in relation to animals, plants, and the world of nature.

9. Play. Being able to laugh, to play, to enjoy recreational activities.

10. Control over one's environment: Political. Being able to participate effectively in political choices that govern one's life; having the right of political participation, protections of free speech and association. Material. Being able to hold property (both land and movable goods), and having property rights on an equal basis with others; having the right to seek employment on an equal basis with others; having the freedom from unwarranted search and seizure. In work, being able to work as a human, exercising practical reason and entering into meaningful relationships of mutual recognition with other workers (Nussbaum, 2000, p.78).

The articulation of ten central capabilities is where Sen and Nussbaum differ in their approaches. Sen prefers the framework to be underspecified to have the broadest possible applications. Nussbaum (2006) believes that each of the ten human capabilities must be met to a sufficient level. Anything less is not a life as a "truly human being" (p. 78). Furthermore, her emphasis on dignity means not exchanging or replacing any of the ten capabilities. Dignity is interactional, between the individual's freedom to choose from a personally meaningful capability set, and importantly, societal contexts that promote such freedoms.

Even when an individual has no meaningful sense of the listed capabilities, Nussbaum maintains that society must strive to offer as many of the capabilities as possible, directly or through a suitable alternative arrangement. The complexity and diversity of disability make this a challenging assertion. For example, significant health disabilities might in extreme circumstances call into question the desire or ability to live a long life. Significant intellectual and developmental disabilities may complicate access to hold property, secure employment on an equal basis with others, or as the primary focus of this book, establish life plans. All human capabilities are relevant to consider within this research.

A Capability Framing

Significantly impacted by disability In one sense, the term *significant disability* is uncomplicated. Within the school setting, those with severe, profound, and multiple disabilities are delineated as being within the highest 3% (in ANZ) or 1% (in USA) of students most severely impacted by their disabilities. While quantified thresholds are clear, they do not clarify the lived realities of severe and complex needs. Nor are they a strengths-based or a capability-oriented way to define disability.

In another sense, the term significant disability is both contentious and vague. Return first to medical and social models of disability used in the previous chapter to understand the implementation of disability practices in the USA and ANZ respectively. Medical conceptions in USA provide individually tailored interventions to address their perceived limitations, while social welfare in ANZ aligns with the UNCRPD to broadly uphold the fundamental human rights of people with disability. Both models are not without critique, however. The medical model can be accused of being overly deficit-oriented, focused on cures, and lacking the complexity and multi-directional dynamics of disability experiences. Comparatively, the social model runs the risk of minimizing individual realities as well as creating an uncomfortable dynamic between those with and without disabilities. The relationship between medical and social models also unnecessarily creates a binary or dichotomy that leads to the question, "where does impairment end and disability start?" (Shakespeare, 2018, p. 127).

Conceptualizing disability is crucial because the way people think about disability impacts how they react to it. Both medical and social models can be brought together in combination when capability is used to define disability. A capability-oriented framing of disability also invites the impacts of other models, such as economic and cultural models, to create a multifaceted understanding of a person's experience. Through a lens of capability, disability is the result of a combination of different factors, such as the nature of an impairment and other personal characteristics (e.g., age, gender, race), the resources available to the individual, and their environment (Mitra, 2006). This is of particular importance to those with non-visible disabilities that are not immediately apparent, such as chronic mental or physical illnesses that significantly impact activities of daily living.

A unique combination of sensory, behavioral, intellectual, physical, and health can all impact disability experiences in unique ways and to various extents. The capability approach offers a strength-based way to accept abilities before disability. To investigate and articulate issues with assumed competence before ineptitude. Diversity is essential to understanding the disability experience and is key to this work.

Transition A novel way to examine individuals' exit from school into adult life is by the way it impacts an individual's capabilities (Hart et al., 2017). Transition within a capability framing involves genuine opportunities. The outcomes, or functionings, of post-school life are typically hallmarks of a "successful" transition, such as gainful employment, enrollment into post-secondary education, or independent living outside the family home. Framed by capability, these become only one unit for examination. Consequentially, a rich understanding of transition develops based on what individuals can do when they have access to both resources and the autonomy or control of their own dignified life.

Using a gender justice example to illustrate, an unnatural imbalance between genders cannot, according to a capability approach, be addressed by resources alone. Certainly, financial stability can assist women's liberation, but capability emphasizes converting those resources into worthwhile and personally meaningful activities. Therefore, a capability approach to addressing gender justice focuses on opportunities to access education, healthcare, political freedoms (like the right to vote), the ability to work and contribute outside of the home, etc. (Robeyns, 2021). Having money and resources will assist these opportunities, but cannot alone secure improved well-being. Continuing the example further, a woman might win the lottery, but if she can't think and reason in a way that is "informed and cultivated by an adequate education" (Nussbaum, 2000, p. 78), then she won't necessarily be prepared to spend this money wisely. Furthermore, if cultural restrictions mean that this lottery money needs to be administrated by a male executor, then she has lost the freedom to apply the funds in her own best interests.

These examples are not meant to oversimplify a vast area of scholarship on capability's contribution to gender justice. Rather, examples are used to situate understanding from outside the central topic of transition. Transition-related injustices will be presented and analyzed extensively in subsequent chapters. In sum, applying the capability approach to post-school transition is not intended to ignore or erase the challenges associated with this critical life stage. Rather, this approach can be used to pinpoint where problems lie when understood directly from the experiences of those with disabilities. Then, new ways to support can be considered. The capability set of those with significant disabilities is thus far more than just access to services and social welfare.

Method of international comparison Returning to its foundations, capability was designed to be used as a measure to compare international human development. The Human Development Index (HDI) used by the United Nations was created based on Sen's articulation of the capability approach. The core of the HDI emphasizes that people and their capabilities should be the ultimate criteria for assessing the development of a country, not economic growth alone. Key dimensions of human development, such as a long and healthy life, being knowledgeable, and having a decent standard of living provide a fuller picture of a country's level of human development (United Nations, 2023).

To give a thorough consideration of post-school transition opportunities, the comparative transition policies described in the prior chapter were examined for their impact on the well-being or freedom that young adults with disabilities have within each country. Also, operational specifications explain how different policy choices yield comparatively different impacts. Sen importantly noted that the capability approach was not designed to provide a utopian ideal, but rather help in making comparisons of injustice, and to guide toward a less unjust society. This work therefore uses a capability frame to examine the opportunity of dignity within transition.

CHAPTER CONCLUSION

Dignity is a key term of capability, used to focus attention to the well-being of every individual in their own right, regardless of ability or disability (Nussbaum, 2006). A central distinction of the capability approach is the establishment of a life of personal value by way of (a) capabilities, what a person can do, be, and finds personally meaningful; (b) freedom, a person's actual opportunities to select from personally relevant opportunities that form an individual's capability set; and (c) functionings, the "beings and doings" (Sen, 1999, p. 6) and realized choices of a person's life. A novel way to examine individuals' exit from school to adult life is by defining transition as the way it expands an individual's capabilities (Hart et al., 2017). A capability frame was used to examine the opportunity of dignity within transition.

REFERENCES

Hart, S. M., Gaffney, J. S., & Hill, M. F. (2017). Critical reflections on emancipatory partnerships in transition research: Discerning perspectives of New Zealand Students on the autism spectrum. *Disability and Society, 32*(6), 831–852. https://doi.org/10.1080/09687599.2017.1329710

Mitra, S. (2006). The capability approach and disability. *Journal of Disability Policy Studies, 16*(4), 236–247. https://doi.org/10.1177/10442073060160040501

Nussbaum, M. C. (2000). *Women and human development: The capabilities approach*. Cambridge University Press.

Nussbaum, M. C. (2006). *Frontiers of justice: Disability, nationality, species membership*. Harvard University Press.

Robeyns, I. (2021). *Wellbeing, freedom, and social justice: The capability approach re-examined*. Open Book Publishers. Retrieved from: https://socialsci.libretexts.org/Bookshelves/Sociology/Cultural_Sociology_and_Social_Problems/Wellbeing_Freedom_and_Social_Justice%3A_The_Capability_Approach_Re-Examined_(Robeyns)

Sen, A. (1999). *Development as freedom*. Oxford University Press.

Shakespeare, T. (2018). *Disability: The basics*. Routledge.

United Nations. (2023). *Human Development Index (HDI)*. Published online at OurWorldInData.org. Retrieved from: https://ourworldindata.org/human-development-index

CHAPTER 4

Methods of Inquiry

Abstract In this chapter, inclusive, qualitative data collection procedures will be described. In Aotearoa New Zealand, an innovative agentic ethnography was implemented. In the USA, a novel technique was employed to create a composite narrative case study from a secondary analysis of the American Voices Project dataset. Ethical research recruitment procedures and data analyses will also be described as they occurred within each study setting. Methodological transparency supports the trustworthiness of the findings presented in subsequent chapters.

Keywords Agentic ethnography • Composite narrative case study • Inclusive research

The research presented in this book is organized around a guiding principle that knowledge about individuals with severe and complex needs must be gained through their active participation and inclusion. When this occurs, novel understandings of transition can be gained and applied to research, praxis, and wider society. Pursuant to these aims, multiple research threads are joined together between countries and social time points through the following research questions: (a) What are the perceptions and meanings of post-school transition experiences for young adults with disabilities, and (b) what are the impacts of these perspectives on how transition can be implemented with dignity?

© The Author(s), under exclusive license to Springer Nature   33
Singapore Pte Ltd. 2024
S. M. Hart, *Transition with Dignity*,
https://doi.org/10.1007/978-981-97-2351-5_4

INCLUSIVE METHODS

The studies conducted in both ANZ and USA were designed to be inclusive, qualitative research. While disability is the focus here, inclusive research is conceptually broad with the overall aim to build a supportive culture for any underrepresented group to participate. Inclusive research is of vital importance for those with disabilities, especially those with more significant disabilities, to break assumptions that such individuals have nothing to say, and so in turn, few listen. All vital components to social belonging and citizenship (Taylor, 2018).

Practically speaking, inclusive research has a wide variety of applications that will be specifically described within each setting. First, however, is a brief description of the unique human research ethics procedures and approaches to invite participation. Namely the nuanced distinction between informed consent and assent. Informed consent is a legal obligation to ensure potential participants enter research voluntarily with full information about what it means for them to take part. Assent should share all the same elements as informed consent, yet it pertains to those who require extra care or consideration (Hart, 2021). During the assent procedures in ANZ, for example, all participant information materials were provided in a manner suitable to the cognitive levels and communication preferences of potential participants. This involved extended time getting to know the young adults and their support networks so that informed assent modifications could be individually tailored. Those research procedures were formally reviewed and approved by the human participants ethics committee (reference number 9727). Informed consent and individually adapted assent procedures were extensively conducted over an extended seven-week period and are described in detail in the publication Hart et al. (2017). In USA, an institutional review was conducted and approved (proposal ID #22-05-056) in order to access sensitive information within the American Voices Project dataset.

AGENTIC ETHNOGRAPHY: DATA COLLECTION IN ANZ

Research in ANZ began within two urban special schools specifically for students with disabilities. Special schools were prioritized, (a) to access a potential participant pool of those with the most significant disabilities, (b) since ANZ does not require students to have a specific disability label to receive services, special schools afforded access to the relevant population, and (c) due to my insider access and understanding as a former special educator. Each selected school was in a setting known for having students with high levels of diversity located in mostly middle to low-socio-economic-status communities (as noted through decile ratings from 1 to 10 indicating the socio-economic makeup of the community). Senior management of the schools managed participant recruitment.

Three individuals and their families volunteered to take part in this study, and ethical consent/assent procedures were conducted as described above. Fieldwork qualitatively captured these cases over six months by tracking progression from in-school to post-school for each young adult in transition. *Agentic ethnography* is the phrase coined to represent how classic ethnographic techniques were inclusively adapted to the communication preferences of the young adult participants, even when some used no verbal communication to express their perspectives (Hart, 2022). Inquiry was directly aligned with each transition as it was experienced by the young adults in real time. Data collection involved: (a) participant observation once per week for each case lasting between one and three hours each session for a total of 103 hours across settings in-school (e.g. classroom, graduation, work experience) and post-school (e.g. community day program, post-secondary education) including associated field notes; (b) semi-structured interviews ($n = 17$) conducted, audio-recorded, and transcribed with transition informants who were classified as having high-influence on transition decisions; and (c) artifact collection ($n = 226$), including photographs, video, and documents collected in-school (e.g. school reports, behavior management plans) and post-school (e.g. funding applications, transition portfolios). When interviews were silent or inconsistently verbal, photographs, and videos were used to record responses. Each adapted interview format was co-constructed through *emancipatory partnerships,* meaning that the focus on the young adults' perspectives outweighed all other contributions to understanding transition (Hart et al., 2017). Adapted techniques ranged from participatory photographic adapted interviews, to context-setting-based interviews, to visual symbol exchanges (for more detailed descriptions of each adapted qualitative technique, please see Hart et al., 2017).

Both inductive and deductive data analyses occurred. First, NVivo analytic software was used to review and inductively code the data corpus in its entirety. Patterns in the codes were initially noted within individual cases and were then merged into overarching themes across the cases. An additional round of deductive analysis was then directly guided by the perspectives of the case participants using the capability approach as a framework. The data corpus was examined for each of the ten central human capabilities (Nussbaum, 2006). Through multiple rounds of interviewing, each participant could raise, clarify, and add depth using the ten central capabilities as analytical guideposts. This process revealed individual capabilities that may have been otherwise overlooked or not raised during the lived experiences of leaving school.

All aspects of the project, from conception, design, and execution, to analysis, proceeded with reflexive researcher consultation, as this study was conducted as part of doctoral study, and then collaboratively disseminated through academic conferences and research journals. The doctoral supervision process allowed for "investigator triangulation" (Brantlinger et al., 2005, p. 199), which ensured a rigorous research design and that interpretations of findings were not idiosyncratic to one personal perspective. Additionally, all finding themes were put into plain language, sign language, and visual symbols. The linguistic formats best suited the communication abilities of the young adults whose transitions had been followed and enabled their ability to review and provide feedback. Data collection measures culminated in prolonged and substantive field engagement recorded in an audit trail that documented the chronology and the amount of time spent at each stage of fieldwork.

AMERICAN VOICES PROJECT: DATASET IN USA

In USA, data came from a secondary analysis of the American Voices Project (AVP) qualitative dataset. This ongoing project created the country's first nationally representative sample of over 2700 interviews through a joint initiative of Stanford and Princeton Universities. Interviews began during the distinctive time period of the Covid pandemic lockdowns.

Through an application and vetting process, approval was granted to access 1613 interview transcripts of the AVP dataset and receive associated technical and research support. All AVP interviews were structured using the same interview probes and lasted approximately three hours each.

Interview transcriptions were provided by AVP within a secured remote server and demographic data was provided within a comprehensive spreadsheet.

A subpopulation of 12 AVP interviews were selected for secondary analysis. These interviews pertained to those within a young adult age range (18–30 years old) who received disability-specific social welfare benefits (Social Security Disability Insurance, SSDI). Secondary analysis involved individually reviewing each participant interview by systematically categorizing themed patterns within individual transcriptions. Extensive transcription quotes were kept intact and analytical memos were made to detail each emergent code. Individual experiences, realities, and responses ranged broadly. The raw and real humanity of the participants' experiences was retained to the greatest extent possible during analysis.

The AVP provided transcription data that was cleansed to remove names and setting details. The AVP's data nondisclosure agreement, however, erred on the side of caution where, amongst other concerns, direct quotes were acceptable for release, yet some information could unintentionally eventuate in re-identification. For example, AVP participation held significant attention within certain small and remote communities, which could re-identify people or conditions within those areas. Furthermore, sensitivity was needed for the differing supports and care that were regionally specific during the pandemic. A composite narrative case method (Willis, 2019) was therefore employed to best adhere to and address the general principles of the AVP disclosure avoidance policy for research intended for publication.

A single convergent and coherent case was constructed from the overlap found between the 12 analyzed AVP cases, referred to here as a *composite narrative case*. Implementing this relatively new method, a first-person account was written as a vignette using multiple data points to represent specific aspects of the research findings (Johnston et al., 2023). The richness, complexity, and situatedness of personal perspectives was kept intact while ensuring the ethical priority of anonymity.

From an audit trail of more than 24 pages of single-spaced text that included direct and indirect transcription quotes and analytical memos (over 12,000 words), a single case was constructed using direct participants' language. Decisions about the demographic details of the composite case were taken from the most common of the 1275 variables collected by AVP through their descriptive statistical analysis (e.g., mean, median, mode) as well as data crosswalks provided (e.g., life aspects such as annual earnings, gender, weeks worked, and expenses). The chronology of in-school to post-school life determined the narrative arc of this transition story. Some minor additions and changes were edited to develop flow and readability, but otherwise, the composite case included quotes and para-phrasing directly from the interview transcripts to depict the central find-ings of the analysis.

As a measure of quality control, the qualitative research technique of *member checking*, also known as participant or respondent validation, was employed (Brantlinger et al., 2005). Broadly speaking, this process involved returning the central findings depicted within the composite case to relevant individuals in the disability community to check for accuracy and resonance with their experiences. The challenge, however, was that the composite case was constructed through secondary data, so original participants could not be part of this member check process. Therefore, pre-service and in-service teachers were employed as research assistants who accessed their personal disability networks to recruit this feedback. Each research assistant was responsible for discussing one research theme. These member checks were conducted via a remote online platform. While those in the disability networks may not have resonated with all aspects of the composite case, this external feedback process was an essential way to ensure truthful accuracy in creating the composite narrative case.

Presentation of Findings

The findings from these described methods will be presented in a few ways. In Chap. 5, case narratives from each country (3 in ANZ, 1 in USA) depict the lived experiences and transition perspectives of young adults (all names are pseudonyms). Each case is joined through a tangible marker of time that is presented chronologically. The narratives consider not only the realities of post-school transition, but also how capability can be used to consider new, and oftentimes more dignified, opportunities. Importantly, the cases of transition were not selected for being exemplary in any sense. In ANZ, ordinary transition cases were selected for their willingness to be studied during this tumultuous life stage. In USA, transition was not the sole or specific focus of AVP interview questions, thus the amalgamated narrative is a composite experience of transition during the specific time-point of the pandemic.

Findings are put forward to prioritize possibility over problems and opportunities over outcomes, as directly aligned with a capability framing. The possibilities of what transition can be will be brought to the fore, and given much needed exploration and consideration. In doing so, this study was not problem-based research, as is most common, but rather possibility-based (Gaffney, 2013).

Through the lens of capability, Chap. 6 liberates readers from being bound to one specific context and is intended to open new considerations for transition policies, practices, and research. It will not, however, rank or prescribe one country's practices over another's. Chapter 6 begins by presenting a capability symbol or metaphor. Each was assigned by me as the researcher/author for their ability to anchor a tangible understanding of transition. Metaphors have a noteworthy history in their contribution to scholarly endeavors (e.g., Lakoff & Johnson, 2008). Each symbol serves as an artifact of transition featured for its situatedness and lived properties. As such, findings are portrayed in scholarly and concrete manners to be relatable to diverse audiences of those with and without disabilities alike.

CHAPTER CONCLUSION

The methods described in this chapter would not have been possible without belief in human capability, that every human being, by virtue of their humanity, has a story (or data) to share. In this sense, the best way to evaluate the research methods and findings is for their abilities to be "informative as well as transformative" (Barton, 2005, p. 318). This methods chapter has described a range of inclusive research innovations in ANZ (agentic ethnography) and USA (composite narrative case study). Ethical research recruitment procedures and data analyses were also described for the cases within each country. Methodological transparency supports the trustworthiness of the findings presented in subsequent chapters.

REFERENCES

Barton, L. (2005). Emancipatory research and disabled people: Some observations and questions. *Educational Review, 57*(3), 317–327. https://doi.org/10.1080/00131910500149325

Brantlinger, E., Jimenez, R., Klingner, J., Pugach, M., & Richardson, V. (2005). Qualitative studies in special education. *Exceptional Children, 71*(2), 195–207. https://doi.org/10.1177/001440290507100205

Gaffney, J. S. (2013, September). Agency in literacy learning (ALL): Possibility-driven research. In *Inaugural Professor Lecture at the Faculty of Education*. University of Auckland.

Hart, S. M. (September 2021). *Diverse voices on disability advocacy during the pandemic in the US. Breaking Boundaries – (Counter) Accounts during the Pandemic*. Open Access Collection.

Hart, S. M. (2022). Agentic ethnography: Methods, positionality, and perspectives of individuals with significant disabilities on the transition from school. *International Journal of Research and Method in Education, 45*(1), 3–17. https://doi.org/10.1080/1743727X.2021.1881057

Hart, S. M., Gaffney, J. S., & Hill, M. F. (2017). Critical reflections on emancipatory partnerships in transition research: Discerning perspectives of New Zealand Students on the autism spectrum. *Disability and Society, 32*(6), 831–852. https://doi.org/10.1080/09687599.2017.1329710

Johnston, O., Wildy, H., & Shand, J. (2023). Student voices that resonate: Constructing composite narratives that represent students' classroom experiences. *Qualitative Research, 23*(1), 108–124. https://doi.org/10.1177/14687941211016158

Lakoff, G., & Johnson, M. (2008). *Metaphors we live by*. University of Chicago Press.

Nussbaum, M. C. (2006). *Frontiers of justice: Disability, nationality, species membership*. Harvard University Press.

Taylor, A. (2018). Knowledge citizens? Intellectual disability and the production of social meanings within educational research. *Harvard Educational Review, 88*(1), 1–25. https://doi.org/10.17763/1943-5045-88.1.1

Willis, R. (2019). The use of composite narratives to present interview findings. *Qualitative Research, 19*(4), 471–480. https://doi.org/10.1177/1468794118787711

Lived Experiences: International Narratives of Transition

Abstract At the central heart of this work, this chapter presents four vividly described narrative portraits of post-school transition. Set in two different countries, each case depicts lived disability experiences in young adulthood.

Keywords Artifacts • Lived experience • Narrative portraits • Timetable • Young adults

Recall that each transition was captured in real time, as it unfolded and naturalistically occurred. This methodological decision was intentional either (a) due to the severity of young adult's disabilities, as was the case in ANZ—these young adults could not reliably reflect or offer preferences about historical aspects of their transitions; or (b), in the case of USA, data was aggregated from an already existing dataset, so no follow-up reflections could be ascertained.

Consequently, a few implications should be mentioned based on these data collection procedures. First, while each narrative belongs to a young person, as a qualitative researcher, I am still part of the research process. I have attempted to stay true to the transitions I understood them, but my prior experiences, assumptions, and beliefs are always present (Bengtsson, 2016). My research presence is mitigated (a) by situating my positionality in prior chapters, (b) by providing extensive descriptions of data collection

S. M. Hart, *Transition with Dignity*,
https://doi.org/10.1007/978-981-97-2351-5_5

procedures, and (c) by the thick and rich details within each case narrative portrait. Second, note that the point-of-view perspective of writing will shift in the chapter; from third-person fieldwork data in ANZ, to a first-person composite interview account in USA. Use of the personal pronoun "I" is an important feature of composite narrative case study as this language indicates that the composite-informant is someone who typifies the general experience, as well as exists within a situated context (Johnston et al., 2023). Third, note that the narrative cases occurred during different time points. The transitions in ANZ were collected approximately five years before the pandemic, whereas the composite case in USA occurred during the pandemic-related lockdowns. A final implication serves as a forewarning to the reader that not all the transition experiences depicted within these cases were optimistic. While the chapter following will analyze transition through the lens of dignity, the focus here is on the raw, complex, and oftentimes messy experiences of leaving school and embarking on young adult life in the community. Caution that occasional foul language is used within interview transcripts, and a content warning that topics covered will include: physical and emotional abuse including neglect, poverty, law enforcement, abusive relationships, and discrimination.

Aotearoa New Zealand

Figure 5.1 provides an organizing framework for the way each case narrative is described as an amalgamation of in-school and post-school experiences. Note: Symbols denote use (+), or lack thereof (−), of timetables in each setting for each young man. Details from in-school and post-school culminate in understanding the personal perspectives of Haku, Cobain, and Faine (all young men—as is commonly found in the special school autism population). The positive (+) or negative (−) notations next to each name refer to whether or not a consistent and meaningful transition timetable artifact was used during that particular transition stage.

A timetable is meant here as a schedule, diary, organizer, or calendar; a way of organizing and structuring within and between days and activities. Use of this artifact was raised by the young man, Faine, and was then consistently found across cases. Each timetable looked different and was used (or not used) in idiosyncratic ways. Timetables served as a pragmatic, tangible lens through which each young adult presented and understood their own transitions. Description of transition-related activities show, on

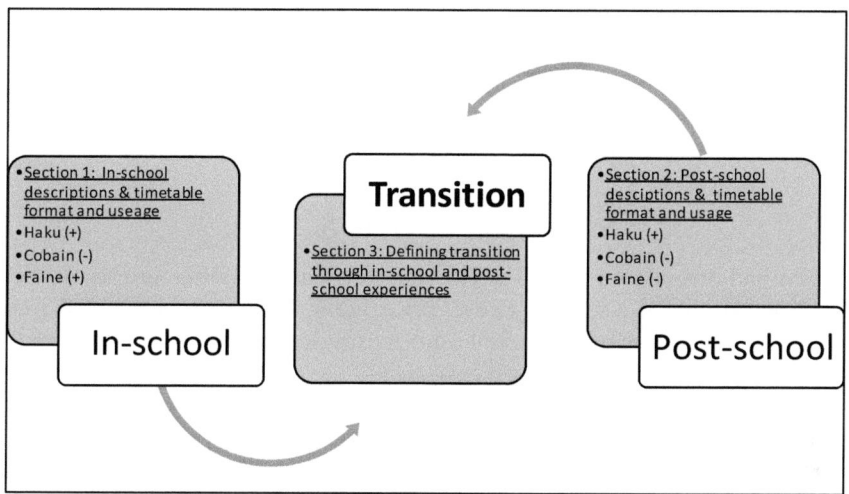

Fig. 5.1 Structure of each case narrative

the surface, activities enjoyed and the nature and frequency with which each engaged in those activities. On a deeper level, theoretically framed by capability, timetables showed potential functionings. They enabled each young person to communicate their knowledge and apply understandings toward post-school futures. Timetables in and of themselves may seem a small, limited item, but their implications will be shown to be far-reaching (Hart et al., 2021).

Haku

Haku was a mild-mannered, sweet young man who spoke verbally, yet mostly using echolalia, repeating back what was already said to him. For him, actions spoke louder than words. His preference was to work visually. He offered his opinions and expressed complex ideas in writing and through art such as drawings and dance. Haku's mother immigrated to ANZ from Japan before Haku was born. She raised Haku on her own. When Haku began school (at age 5 in ANZ), his mother reported knowing nothing about special schools. Due to her son's disabilities, she was strongly encouraged by a disability support person (possibly a medical professional) that her son should attend such a school. His hobbies included playing video games, reading magazines about video games, and participating in drama and dance. Haku moved from strength to strength in his transition. Evidence is used to demonstrate positive experiences in both in-school and post-school settings. Correspondingly, the timetable Haku used successfully in both environments will be described.

SECTION 1: HAKU IN SCHOOL

Haku had attended a school exclusively for students with significant disabilities, known as a special school, since age 5. In an interview, he shared the following views of his special school experiences,

Haku: [School name] means to be special school. And we get some to the *special people and autistic and artistic.*
Sarah: Interesting! What are special people?
Haku: It's getting, wandering around people and also maybe …
Sarah: This is very good, Haku. Please tell me more.
Haku: Special school is the special needs and she's gonna help us, teacher aides and teachers. *Special school helps us and special needs and teachers and teacher aides.* (Interview transcript, Haku, in-school phase, emphasis added)

In this extract, keywords are italicized to show how Haku expressed his understanding of special school in his own words. He unpacked central features of special-school life: help and support from teachers, paraprofessional teaching assistants (also called teacher aides), and students who have both disability and capability, "autistic and artistic." Haku was unable to verbally compare special schools to mainstream educational environments. Through a photographic interview, however, he visually identified some features that made his class unique. For example, unlike a typical classroom, his classroom contained such things as a video game console with corresponding flat-screen TV and couches. This "senior learning environment" was more akin to an office breakroom, with a kitchenette, computers, and work desks included.

Haku's community-based classroom was a safe, familiar space. In adapted interview he took photographs using a smartphone camera feature. He photographed cupboards and described from memory objects that were found in each. Through photographs, he drew attention to the wall displays that highlighted some of his achievements over the school year. Photos were displayed of his solo dance performance in a disability arts show, using the community gym, and participating in work experience. In this manner, he drew attention to the features of the class curriculum that were important to him. The activities did not appear to be out of the ordinary in relation to his class's curriculum. What stood out were Haku's competencies in the activities he highlighted. He appeared to have a far higher level of mastery than his peers in the examples that he chose to portray.

For instance, at the start of fieldwork, Haku participated in a three-day disability arts festival. Haku's class was performing a dance routine and he enjoyed a central role as a principal solo dancer. Another observed skill of Haku's was in the community gym. Haku and a male classmate independently managed their entire visit to the gym. They walked to the gym from their community-based classroom, used a gym tag to sign in, put their gym bags away in the locker room, then stretched and used weight and cardio training machines. Both young men used a visual booklet with photographs made by their teachers to guide their gym routine. Haku referred to his dutifully, while his classmate followed Haku's lead.

A central feature in the classroom display of successful accomplishments was Haku's work experience. Haku worked unpaid, three hours per week at a building supply store. Staff from school dropped him off and picked him up. In the past, staff had to support Haku at the employment site. He had been doing the job for two years by the time of observation, so now he worked independently with only the supervision of his boss.

Haku's work experience was fun, even for an observer. Haku had a set work routine, to dust and wipe down the display case at the front of the store, that he had memorized, and he later described a context-led adapted interview. "There's over NZ$200,000 worth of products he's handling on those shelves," his boss explained (Quote transcript, field notes, in-school phase). While Haku worked on his cleaning routine, his boss sat at the front checkout counter greeting and joking with customers. When Haku's boss needed him for an extra errand he yelled loudly, "Captain!" Responding to his nickname, Haku would stop what he was doing, briskly walk up to the checkout counter, and occasionally even salute his boss in a joking fashion, replying, "Yes, Chief!" Haku's one-off tasks included passing messages across the various store departments and assisting in unloading vending machines.

Haku's boss was like a proud father, he bragged about Haku's accomplishments as he worked. "He's strong," his boss observed as he pointed to boxes of nail packaging that Haku stacked for them. Haku chimed in, "that's because I go to the gym." Then the annual store stock take was mentioned. "Nothing wrong with his counting at all! Haku's counts go straight to the head office." Haku wouldn't talk when he first started the job, his boss recalled. "He's come a long way" (Field notes, in-school phase).

When asked in a context-based interview how long he had worked at the building supply store, Haku didn't know. He wanted to have an answer, so he first suggested that he went to work every day. Then his response changed to working at the building supply store for only one month. What he did know, with perfect accuracy, was all of his work colleagues' names. He greeted each of them as they walked into the break room. Likewise, he knew all the power tool names and their manufacturers.

Timetables At the beginning of fieldwork, Haku was observed writing in his timetable. He used an A4-sized hardbound, daily diary to plan, structure, and review each day. Once a week, he glued in a weekly calendar to give an overview of his activities and note any changes in his weekly routines. He knew the procedure well: fill in a blank printout timetable, cut to size, and paste it in on the page. He knew the content of the timetable and activities from memory.

Haku's special-school teacher commented in his end-of-school report,

> Haku continues to write in his diary when he is at school. He uses his time-table to manage his school week and it was lovely to hear of Haku preparing and planning ahead for various school activities without Mum even knowing it was happening. Super management Haku, your weekly timetable is so busy that I am sure you are the only one who knows what is happening each day. Well done! (End-of-Year report, Artifact, in-school phase).

SECTION 2: POST-SCHOOL: POLYTECHNIC

When Haku finished school, he transitioned into a polytechnic program akin to a trade school. The program included coursework specifically designed for students with disability to learn general pre-employment skills, rather than develop a specific trade. As a prerequisite, he had attended a one-day-a-week course during the final semester at school. The polytechnic curriculum was geared toward students who held few or no credits[1] from secondary school. The polytechnic course was popular. Approximately 50 new students enrolled each year, coming from suburbs across the city.

In one of the two observed transition planning meetings, the transition team discussed the full-time nature of the polytechnic program: from 9:00 am to 3:00 pm, five days a week. During the meeting, Haku spoke up and noted that he wanted to remain working at the building supply store. There had been an assumption he would finish his work experience to attend polytechnic full time. The team scrambled to consider how they might be able to accommodate Haku's request.

Following the meeting, and again in a social media post, Haku's mother expressed surprise at her son's assertiveness in the meeting. He typically never spoke unless directly asked a question. She knew if her son expressed an interest in his work experience, it was important to him, and she called upon his transition coordinator to make this happen for her son. Haku's boss was happy for him to continue and the polytechnic program teachers agreed and permitted Haku to miss one morning a week to work.

Haku's first day in the polytechnic was as stereotypical as any first day imaginable. He took a campus tour and was then issued a student ID. Upon reflection, the most salient observation was how this day was possibly the most inclusive of Haku's polytechnic experience. All other observations were held on a segregated part of campus in classrooms designated only for students in this disability-specific, pre-employment program. The only opportunities for inclusion within mainstream campus activity were at lunchtimes when students had the option to eat at one of the campus cafes. Haku was never observed to choose this option. He preferred to eat lunch in the polytechnic program's staff room, an option available to, and commonly used by, many of his classmates.

Once the polytechnic program was underway, an observation was conducted during a mathematics lesson. The class of 56 students was broken into small groups. Each group was responsible for transferring an image from paper onto the sidewalk by following a grid pattern. Haku was very good at this task and did most of the sidewalk chalk drawing. Two of Haku's peers photographed as they watched the group's work. These two

---

[1] New Zealand's National Certificate of Educational Achievement (NCEA) is the national qualification for senior secondary school students. NCEA and the related national certificates are used as benchmarks for selection into university, polytechnics, and employment.

students had physical disabilities that prevented them from getting to and from the ground, mobility that was required to complete this activity.

After the mathematics lesson, an interview was held with the lead polytechnic teacher. The lead teacher said she often found students from special schools to be very well prepared for the pre-employment program at the polytechnic, yet there were not many who attended. Haku was one of only two students in the polytechnic program who had previously attended a special school. He was quite resilient to attend the polytechnic with no social connections when he arrived. The lead teacher mentioned his coping skills: "In computing class, he knows to sit next to two students who *have it* and he can watch and follow them" (Quote transcription, field notes, post-school phase).

The teacher then described students who more commonly enroll at the polytechnic. She pointed out one young woman who had come from a fully inclusive secondary school experience. The young woman struggled to adjust to the disability-specific polytechnic program because she had never realized until now that she in fact had a disability. The teacher then indicated another student, a young man who had Down syndrome, with the best reading comprehension she'd ever taught. The teacher noted there were no other places for him to go after secondary school. He had academic abilities beyond his peers in the pre-employment course, but not enough credits to enroll in other post-secondary education options. The lead teacher said she constantly grappled with how segregated her students were from the rest of the polytechnic campus, yet she wasn't aware of any other alternatives.

Timetable On the first day at the polytechnic, a free orientation tote bag was issued to each student. Among other items in the bag was a diary in the same format as the one Haku had used while in school. It was noted by the lead teacher that the diary would be used throughout the year, so classmates should put their names and contact details inside.

During the next polytechnic observation, Haku's class had a free half hour that they used to finish a previous assignment worksheet activity. As described in field notes:

> The procedure of writing in his visual diary had now become second nature to Haku. The teacher handed out a slip of paper asking the students to describe the lesson in one word. She collected the words anonymously and comments included, "fun and happy." "Good-ish," was Haku's word. The

student next to Haku asked for help on spelling *excited* and mistook *d for b.*
Another student used a dictionary to spell her word. (Field notes, post-
school phase)

Section 3: Transition

When assessed by the consistent diary timetable format, Haku's movement into polytechnic went seamlessly. Through consistent diary use in
in-school and post-school contexts, Haku could set out his week, note any
changes to schedule, and plan for upcoming activities (e.g., budget, list
items to bring). He could also use the diary to debrief on how activities
went, as described in the field notes from the polytechnic. Haku transitioned from what was acknowledged to be masterful use of his timetable
in special school, to have the same confidence in using his timetable at the
polytechnic.

Interestingly, this consistency in timetable use was serendipitous, not
planned. All polytechnic students (institution-wide, not solely the students in the disability-specific pre-employment course) were issued a diary.
It was purely a coincidence that Haku used the same timetable structure
in both school and post-secondary environments. Timetables were personally meaningful, individualized, and served as a daily anchor that provided consistency and stability during a challenging time of life.

Cobain

Cobain lived in care support residences since his tenth birthday. His
mother struggled with her son's living situation but noted that the family,
including his younger brother, felt Cobain's care needs had dominated
their family's life. In addition to being profoundly impacted by autism,
Cobain had significant intellectual disability and had not fully learned to
toilet himself. He also had a vision impairment his mother described as like
"seeing through Swiss cheese" (Interview transcript, Cobain's mother, in-
school phase). Cobain did not speak verbally and had occasional aggressive behaviors such as biting and pinching, which seemed to arise from
nowhere. Cobain attended special school since age five. He was of Pākehā
origins, a New Zealand Māori term for someone of white, typically
European background. Cobain enjoyed music, food, and sensory stimula-
tions such as shadows, the noise from a dehumidifier, and crumpled paper.
His transition story is a hard one to tell. He experienced obstacles in both
in-school and post-school environments. His narrative chronicles those
challenges.

SECTION 1: COBAIN IN SCHOOL

When asked for a tour around his school, Cobain went to hiding places away from the action—places like under picnic tables, behind couches, and at the front door. One of the calmest places was the olive grove. Cobain sat beside olive trees, relaxing, and lying on his back. He got there without the use of his white cane walking stick for support. His teaching staff commented that he enjoyed the shadows made by the trees, though he only went to the olive grove occasionally. The weather was not particularly sunny on this specific day. Cobain's gestures seemed to indicate that he was intentionally demonstrating something special for the sake of the observation.

Music lessons were another setting for observation. Sessions were structured in two half-hour blocks, once per week. The class was split into the "quiet" students, who had a relaxing music session, and the "loud" students, who played the drums and more active music. Cobain was in the former group. After the session, his music teacher was interviewed. She reported her opinion that Cobain was not his usual self during this observation. It was speculated that the loud noise of the lawn mower outside that day may have caused distraction. Yet, there were still evident elements of Cobain's enjoyment of music class. For example, she pointed out his finger tapping to the beat of the music and following the harmonica as the teacher moved around the room making music.

Music class offered a structured routine that engaged Cobain's interest. In music, he was considered capable and was expected to contribute to the music session in his way. Music was, however, atypical in terms of the experiences observed during his time in school. His teacher described during the first classroom observation,

> Cobain doesn't quite belong to the class. He can get up and go whenever he wants. He can join. He doesn't have to join. He doesn't have to sit at the table if he doesn't want to …. He does not like being part of a group. So when *they* [his transition team] start, that's going to be fun to watch. (Interview transcript, in-school phase)

This quote revealed a few crucial points. First and most strikingly, it was the final term at the end of Cobain's time at school, yet his teacher believed his transition was yet to begin. Furthermore, it was anticipated that finding a suitable post-school plan would be challenging. Second, the teacher's use of the word "they" in her quote implied she didn't feel she was included as a part of his transition. Third, she had already moved on from Cobain being her student. She had taught Cobain for years. Some of those years, she reported, were very positive. At this final stage of his education, she had no expectations left for him. He didn't quite "belong" to her class.

In contrast to the music lesson, most of Cobain's in-school observations resembled the following experience from a week before his graduation. On this occasion, all doors in the school were locked from classroom to school entry doors. This was done to reduce the possibility that a student who was experiencing frequent aggressive outbursts would target more vulnerable students. There was one female student who was specifically being targeted. In Cobain's classroom, a male classmate was shouting and rocking. Twice he stripped himself naked. On another two attempts, he failed due to quick staff intervention. Cobain's teacher pronounced in front of the whole class that she wanted to quit.

Amongst the chaos surrounding him, Cobain was in a pleasant mood. Staff were doing their best to calm students and address the misbehaviors of their peers. Certainly, these large and loud behaviors hindered the ability to teach any set curriculum. Thus, the time with Cobain was used to hold the second of two object-exchange interviews, which require a brief background description.

Previously, cues in Cobain's object-cue timetable were used as adapted interview probes. The idea behind the object-cue timetable was that the object-cues served as prompts, representative of the upcoming activity. For example, in the case of the previously described music lesson, were the timetable used, Cobain could have felt a small maraca on a wooden shelf, taken it, and used the maraca as part of the music session. When Cobain returned to the classroom after music, he would feel an empty shelf where the music maraca had formerly been placed, then feel the next shelf down indicating the next activity. A spoon could indicate it was time for lunch, the activity following music. In the first adapted interview, Cobain seemed unsure of the novel interview format and possibly distracted by the sensory stimulation of the sun reflecting on the metal spoon object-cue.

Without observing the timetable in use, a random sampling of object cue activity prompts were presented to Cobain—a small scrap of cloth (symbolism unknown), a spoon (lunch), and measuring cup (cooking). Each item was rustled to make a sound, and after a short time, Cobain pulled out the cloth with a huge smile on his face (photograph recorded, in-school fieldwork phase). In all of his moving around he accidently dropped and lost the cloth. All the items were again presented similarly. He again grabbed the cloth and rustled it to mimic the way it had initially been presented.

From there, a teaching support staff member was asked about the scrap of cloth timetable cue. A regular reliever (substitute) teacher aide (paraprofessional) explained that it was an object cue representing the sensory room. Sensory room activities develop a student's senses, usually through special lighting, music, and objects. It can be used as therapy, oftentimes for those with sensory disabilities and limited communication skills. The same teacher aide described that she was assigned to take Cobain to the sensory room earlier that morning. Yet, as he arrived at the sensory room door, he gestured toward the bathroom. By the time he finished there, he seemed hungry, so they instead went back to class for an early morning tea (snack). This same teaching assistant was also in charge of taking him to the sensory room last week, and reported that he had enjoyed himself. He particularly liked the light reflected on a hanging, white bed sheet and strings that hung down from the ceiling while lit with interchanging different colors. But Cobain hadn't made it to the sensory room on the day of his adapted interview. Cobain overheard this conversation and became so overjoyed that he laid back on the floor with the cloth still in his hand (photograph recorded, in-school fieldwork phase) and kicked his feet back and forth.

Underlying Cobain's final days in special school was the assertion by Cobain's mother that Cobain and his family would not attend his school graduation ceremony. Cobain had a scheduling conflict, with a holiday party at his residential care house on the same day as graduation. While the scheduling conflict was a straightforward explanation for not attending, Cobain's mother was also extremely stressed about her son's graduation. She discussed her emotions in an interview, again in one transition planning meeting, and finally in Cobain's end-of-year report meeting with his teacher.

While observing school graduation, Cobain's mother was ironically one of the first to arrive. Rather than explain what changed her mind, she quickly asserted that she didn't want Cobain to know she was present. She reasoned that if he were to sit with her, he wouldn't want to take part in the graduation ceremony, preferring to stay by her side instead. Or perhaps another interpretation was she already felt exceedingly stressed and didn't want her son to increase the tension. Cobain arrived at graduation with residential care-support staff about 45 minutes late. He struggled to stay in his specially allocated graduation seat on the stage. When he began to walk around on the stage, another graduate's family invited him to sit next to them. Later, in the graduation ceremony, Cobain's father announced they had bought the school an award cup to be named in their son's honor. He made a speech through a teary voice:

> This gives me great pleasure giving this award, it's for my special son. Cobain, love him to death. And I'd like to take this opportunity to thank the school. All the caregivers, all the teachers who have helped Cobain over the years. And anyone else who has helped him grow and made him who he is. Excuse me [as he choked back tears]. (Quote transcript, field notes, in-school phase)

The school was sparsely furnished on Cobain's last day. The teachers had packed up all the furniture, so students sat on the floor or on the few permanent picnic benches outside. Cobain spent his last day at the front door. He didn't try to push, or pinch, or run away. He just stood at the door and waited to leave. A teacher aide mentioned that he'd been there all week. Not long after being dropped off at school, he'd turn around and wait to go home. "He's over it, he's finished [with school]," Cobain's teacher aide reported (Field notes, in-school phase).

Since there were four graduates in Cobain's class, the board of trustees chairperson came to the class to give one final round of congratulations to each of them. Cobain was in the classroom at that moment and moved to sit closer to the chairperson. After a few minutes of sitting near her, he got up and hugged her. She gave him a kiss on the cheek and congratulated him. He smiled and she gave him another kiss. He tensed a bit gesturing to pull her somewhere, but then looked as though he thought better of it. He let go of her hand and went back to the front door.

Cobain's was one of the last taxi transports to arrive at the end of the day. His teacher cried when she said goodbye to most of her graduates. No tears fell for Cobain. The members of the senior management team and the board of trustees chair were at the front door of the school to say goodbye to the graduates. But since Cobain's taxi was late, there was no one left to farewell him.

Timetables Through a successful object-exchange interview with Cobain, it was evident that he understood these tangible artifacts as meaningful and representative of the activities of his day-to-day school life. Since they were never observed in use, it was worthwhile to enquire about the impact of scheduling and routines had on his well-being. With an inability to ask him directly such a line of questions, this understanding was clarified through a re-examination of six occasions where he was observed demonstrating a somewhat calendric capability. This was defined as instances when he exhibited not only knowledge of the upcoming activity but more like an accurate internal clock to know what time the activity would begin. For example,

> It was time for the afternoon "cuppa," cup of tea to end the day. A few students stopped by the table, but Cobain was already sitting at the table before the teapot was even set down. (Field notes, in-school phase)

Not only did Cobain have the ability to know his day-to-day scheduled activities, but he also had an internal understanding of days of the week and even months. This was reported by many who knew him, and comments were sometimes offered as part of other discussions. Many of the conversations were about Cobain's favorite activity, going home to visit his parents:

> Cobain's teacher aide suggested his aggravated behavior at school might be in excited anticipation of going home to his parent's house this evening. She mentioned that they often have difficulties getting him to settle on Mondays for this reason. (Field notes, in-school phase)
>
> Cobain is happy, residential staff explained, because he spent the evening at his parent's house. He showed his joy with a bounce in his step, repeating a "Ha" sound, and occasionally bumping his head into [residential staff's] shoulder or hand. (Video recording, post-school phase)
>
> He knows his routine. He knows what day he comes home. And if I don't have him home for one reason or another, and it has to be something I can't get out of, something major, he'll be shitty the next time he comes home. (Interview transcript, Cobain's mother, in-school phase)

These examples evidence Cobain's calendric capabilities. He knew his routine, and his schedule was important to him. Even though he had a timetable, it was never observed in use during school. Nor were Cobain's calendric abilities observed to be discussed in connection with transition planning or processes.

SECTION 2: POST-SCHOOL: INDIVIDUALIZED COMMUNITY-BASED PROGRAM

Following his transition out of school, Cobain continued to live in the same community-care setting with staff that cared for him and four other young men with special needs of similar ages (akin to a group home). His mother was involved through regular meetings, at which planning for Cobain's community-based activities was discussed. Three planning meetings were observed and occurred at Cobain's residential care home.

Details and reflections about the third and final transition planning meeting serve as an introduction to Cobain's post-school experiences. On this occasion, Cobain's mother was 20 minutes late. Cobain's transition coordinator and residential house leader used the time to talk about how plans for the central feature of his transition program, horseback riding, were still uncertain. Over time, various combinations of Cobain and his teaching team, his mother, and his residential house staff had been to visit a horse, and reports were that typically these visits did not go well. Cobain pulled to return to the car instead of being interested in the horse. They agreed it was not too late for Cobain to enroll in a community day program, at least a few days a week, instead of focusing on horse riding. They also agreed that Cobain's mother was not yet emotionally ready to handle this decision because prior visits to day services had left her upset.

After Cobain's mother arrived, the transition team explained that the purpose of this meeting was a final handover to mark the completion of the transition from school process. Cobain's transition coordinator raised her concerns to the group. For example, about Cobain having a restricted peer group and limited opportunities for a social life now that he had finished school. Her concerns did not gain traction, as conversations fairly quickly went back to tactical decisions about how to make a success of horseback riding.

After the conclusion of the final planning meeting, Cobain's transition provider made an offhand comment using a memorable phrase, "more to life than services." She used the phrase to describe situations like Cobain's where custodial concerns, such as his residential care routines, dominated and suppressed his ability to develop and grow. She was saddened by Cobain's transition. Even with the extensive services available to someone like him with very high needs, aspects of his life were left unaddressed. Cobain had "no room to move" from within the large residential service (Quote transcript, post-school phase).

In the weeks after school had finished, Cobain's mother reported that her son was depressed. He had been crying, banging himself on the head, and not sleeping well. It was hard to get a clear picture of the accuracy of these claims because the comments were made by Cobain's mother and the administrator of the care service. Cobain's house leader, who was involved with his day-to-day care, remained carefully ambiguous about any concerns if she held them. With four other housemates to attend to, logistics and planning of the housemates and care staff took most of her attention.

Four observations were conducted during Cobain's post-school, individualized community-based programs. The description of one observation revealed many of the common features across all observations. In this instance, Cobain and two of his housemates attended an "individualized" adapted arts program held in a community hall.

Before leaving the house, Cobain spent 40 minutes waiting outside for his housemates to be ready to leave in the shared house van transportation. While sitting in the van waiting, Cobain's key support worker described the constant juggle with transportation. Five young men were living in the house, each with individualized programs, and they all needed to share one van. To ease the burden on the shared van, learning to ride public transportation was a prioritized goal for a few of the housemates, including Cobain. Yet, when tried, Cobain refused to get on the bus when it came to the bus stop. While another of his housemates might have been more suited to accessing public transportation, he was "a runner" (Quote transcript, post-school phase). Behavioral issues of absconding made using public transportation too risky because he would spontaneously run far and fast into unsafe conditions. Challenges associated with the housemate's absconding behavior loomed over much of the residential care house. For example, a very loud siren went off every time the front gate was opened to let someone in or out of the house property.

Once the housemates had arrived at the adapted arts class Cobain was observed to engage for only three minutes of the hour-long art session. One of those minutes was a finger painting he made with hand-over-hand support from his house leader, who dipped Cobain's hands into paints and manually spread them onto the paper. The next minute of engagement was bubble paints, where art attendees were meant to blow bubbles through a straw mixed with liquid soap and food coloring onto a page of paper. Cobain drank the bubble mixture. In his final minute of engagement, Cobain was given clean straws to stack and construct with, but he tried to eat them instead.

Cobain spent the remaining 57 minutes of the lesson at the door exit, either lying on the floor or standing at the door. His house leader pulled a large whiteboard in front of the glass doors that led into the common area of the community hall because Cobain kept tapping at the door handle as if to gesturally indicate his interest in leaving. After one door was blocked, Cobain switched to pass time at the other fire exit door (photographs collected, post-school phase). Some of the other housemates were more engaged than Cobain in the art lesson. So even though this was his individualized program, Cobain needed to wait for everyone to be finished.

The class was led by a staff member from another residential care house within the consortium of the care service. All the art class participants had disabilities. This was not a public community class with a diverse range of attendees including those with and without disability. To attend, participants had to pay art supply fees for the term. Cobain's housemate's family paid for the rental of the community hall space. The art class physically took place in a community hall, yet all other aspects of the experience were segregated for only individuals with disability within the residential care service.

Timetable Awareness of Cobain's calendric capabilities was known to his transition team, as highlighted in the prior quotations and examples of his school timetables. Cobain's house leader also demonstrated her awareness of his calendric capabilities following a visit with the Foundation for the Blind, which was described in field notes:

> In Cobain's recent paperwork, his weekly timetable that was arranged by his residential staff was briefly discussed (Artifact collected, day program, post-school phase). Cobain's house leader was excited about her developments with the Foundation for the Blind. Cobain had two visits from a representative of the organization. His house leader showed a picture and described an alarm clock that can announce scheduled activities when set to the specified activity time. Staff would need to remember to stop the stopwatch, otherwise, the clock would keep repeating the audio announcements (Field notes, post-school phase)

By the end of fieldwork, the alarm clock had not eventuated, nor were there any further discussions about its implementation. This is not to assume the alarm clock idea did not happen at some future stage. Even if Cobain did get an audio alarm clock, however, it would have been a new timetable format, one which would require a whole range of new learning. Some such learning might be incompatible with his capability set, as alluded to in the comment about staff having to shut the alarm off for Cobain. Having to learn a new system seemed unnecessary and disruptive to a familiar, though inconsistently used, timetable routine that had already been established in school.

Section 3: Transition

Many disconnects were apparent when applying Cobain's timetable experiences to his transition. First, he had an object-cue timetable procedure that he knew and understood, even though evidence led to an assumption that it was inconsistently, if hardly ever, used during the latter stage of his time in school. Second, transition might have been a time to revisit his existing timetable system, and possibly even used to support Cobain's move between the in-school and post-school environments. This was not done, nor even discussed as an option. Third, an entirely new timetable system was excitedly discussed in a fashion akin to a fun, new gadget, wanting to keep up with technology, but with little regard to Cobain's actual ability to potentially use the timetable independently. The only consistency, sadly, was that despite Cobain's calendric capability and the observed importance of monitoring his time, timetables were not consistently used in his transition.

Faine

Faine lived with his mother, older brother (age 27 at the start of the study), and occasionally with foster children his mother supported. At the start of the study, Faine's mother reported their household had recently gone down from 12 people to four. Faine was of indigenous Māori descent and had a large whānau, an extended family with very close-knit ties. Faine's educational history began in Kura Kaupapa Māori, an immersion Māori language class within a mainstream school. The class ran until his intermediate years (around age 12). Faine had a few years of being home-schooled, then ended up enrolled in a special school that he attended for three years. Until special school, Faine's mother had always been a support teacher in his classes.

Faine was a quiet and content young man, who loved to talk once he got to know you. His mother never sought a formal diagnosis of his disability label, but Faine's educational program indicated he had autism-spectrum-like conditions with related learning disabilities. Faine could not read and write yet enjoyed using the computer to view pictures. He also enjoyed music and was very artistic in media such as drawing, painting, sculpture, and clothing design. While the broad strokes of Faine's transition were straightforward, even though fieldwork afforded insider access to transition events as they unfolded, certain details were never fully clarified. Stories about Faine occasionally took on an exaggerated or even folk tale-like status. For example, everyone from school to family to community members knew Faine had personal capabilities. Yet, for some, Faine's capabilities were so strong they were more like powers beyond typical human ability.

SECTION 1: IN-SCHOOL: FAINE'S SHORT TIME AT SPECIAL SCHOOL

Understanding Faine's educational history is important to his story. Unlike Haku and Cobain, he did not attend special school for his entire educational career. He only attended special school for three years before aging out of school at 21. He would have preferred to stay longer, as occurred at other of his school stages as well. Faine's mother explained her son's educational history in this way,

Faine's mother: What happened was, oh this is a whole story about special ed., but he was in total immersion, Kura, where they just spoke Māori. But the age group stopped at intermediate, about 10 years old at the latest. He came out of three years [in intermediate school] and no one would take him ... He'd just done three years with a group of kids [in intermediate school] and they all knew him. And [the secondary school] up the road wouldn't take him.

Sarah: Was this back in the days when Faine had big antisocial behaviors?

Faine's mother: No, well yeah, but nothing major.

Sarah: So why wouldn't they take him?

Faine's mother: Out of zone, any excuse you can use. Anyway, they choose their students. So we went to [a different secondary school] and couldn't get him in there. He was just horrified. He wanted to stay at the Kura, that's where he wanted to be. So we got an extension for him to go to the Kura and stay there. Which was another hard road. And then [an outreach itinerant teacher from special school] started coming. Faine formed a relationship with [the outreach teacher] and he'd say "come and see my school." And they'd go out for like half a day or something. Then it got a bit longer, then a whole day, to a week. Faine loved [the outreach teacher] and really trusted him. Probably the first person he trusted outside of our family. And that's how he got into special school .... [Outreach teacher] was such a great advocate for Faine. Otherwise, we never would have found special school.

Sarah: So you never thought of a special school sort of route?

Faine's mother: No. I never ever knew they existed. Cause we struggled with mainstream. All by myself. We went on without support [financial or caregiving]. And we kept struggling through. And every time it was time for him to go to another school, I moved a year ahead of him. So when he was at primary I was there all the time. Not with him, but teaching at the school ... So that was our first separation, when he started going to special school. We've been together 24-7 and the three years he's been at special school is the only time we've been separated.

Sarah: It's amazing to me that you work in the school system and yet felt like you didn't know your options.

Faine's mother: I went through all that with no support. I mean he could have had a laptop to work on. Did I know that? No. Now I found out all these things that I never knew that he can't use because he's leaving school. Too old. So I've made it my thing, if there are any others coming through school that they know that special schools are out there. And other schools like that. And becoming aware of all the resources there are. (Faine's mother, interview transcript, in-school phase)

From this passage comes the understandable impression that Faine and his family began his experience at special school hesitantly, after having felt unsupported by social and educational services. His mother never even knew special schools existed. Faine had a history of schools rejecting him.[2]

---

[2] From my understanding, turning down a student from their local school would be illegal, but this is what happened from Faine's mother's perspective. Enrollment in senior schools was not the study focus, so the issue was not pressed for more details.

Faine's reticence to begin special school was also because, at 18 years old, this marked the first time he attended a school separate from where his mother was teaching.

By the time of meeting Faine he was completing special school. The school's Associate Principal described, "I have seen you grow and develop into a wonderful confident young man who has good direction for his future" (End-of-year summary, Associate Principal's comment, in-school phase). Faine's school reports had a long list of accomplishments, such as giving a speech at the opening of his community classroom, being the lead singer in the school band, and holding the role of the school's senior supervisor for their kapa haka cultural group. "From shy Faine to leader Faine in a couple of years. You have helped shape the work and culture of the school" (End-of-year summary, Principal's comment, in-school phase).

Faine's final Individualized Education Plan had goals around leadership and communicating with unfamiliar people. Evidence of his achievements in these areas included, for example, his responsibility for giving the Māori blessing when visitors joined for shared meals at school, and his roles as senior Māori supervisor when new students enrolled. The development of his opportunities to meet and communicate with new people came from social-skills curricular sessions, work experience, visiting the public gym, and community visits to places such as the grocery store.

Faine's work experience was an early fieldwork observation. While at his community-based school classroom, his teacher prompted Faine to get ready for work, and then he prepared himself with a jolt of energy. He brushed his hair, packed his morning tea snack, and put on his uniform t-shirt for the chain store where he worked. As he walked to work with a classmate and teacher aide, Faine cracked jokes about his job. He knew the route to walk to work, and how to clock in on the time clock once he got there. On this occasion, he was working in the garden department. During his work in the garden department, Faine needed help from his teacher aide, which was offered very patiently and supportively, although no independent work skills were being taught. The teacher aide confirmed there were no responsibilities at the department store Faine could do independently. Faine was calm, patient, and focused throughout the observation of his work experience, but showed no signs this would be a job he could do independently in the future as paid work. This was in contrast to his classmate who was working in a different department of the store without teacher support. Yet, this did not deter Faine's morale or the willingness of his teaching team to let him try.

In another fieldwork observation, Faine and half his classmates were preparing for the upcoming school ball (senior school prom) by cooking some simple finger foods. Faine worked with a group of four classmates and contributed by making savory pastries. As described in field notes,

> Faine was clearly the least capable of his group of classmates. He struggled with fine motor coordination to use the knife and to spread the filling onto the pastry and roll it. He seemed aware of his inadequacies and would cover it up by joking with comments like, "My eyes are stinging from onions!" His teachers stuck with him and refused to let him fail. There were no opportunities to give up, just to finish in his way and time. For example, they were okay that his onions were cut to different sizes, and the pastry was rolled in a style unlike the classmates. They didn't care that the final product might have not looked as "polished" as his classmates. For this, Faine remained in good spirits and happily volunteered to help with the dishes. (Field notes, in-school phase)

Adaptions made by teaching staff supported Faine's opportunities to try new things. Faine could feel this support as well, which he demonstrated by not getting discouraged or frustrated. In doing so, he experienced accomplishments throughout school.

A further observation was held at an art studio. This venue was another instance of a physically integrated setting exclusively attended by those with disability (akin to Cobain's experience). Faine was sitting next to two classmates, the teacher aide who supported his work experience, and a young woman not from his school. They were the most talkative of the group of 20 or so artists who sat at long art benches skirting the art room. They laughed and joked about topics only adolescents would find funny, like times they injured themselves. Upon further listening it became apparent the conversation topics were mostly fabricated. For instance, they spoke of when they were joining professional wrestling matches or playing games in their private swimming pool. They also had an amazing repertoire of jokes. For example, Faine knew many pirate jokes—"What's a pirate's favorite singer? Rrrrr Kelly!" The most factual conversation they shared was about music and musician gossip. The conversations at times fell into fiction, when, for example, they took turns listing all the concerts they had attended and the musicians they met afterward. Both Faine and his female classmate demonstrated a good running knowledge of musicians' top hits and upcoming concerts (Field notes, in-school phase).

Faine's mother was outside after art class finished. She worked at a school nearby and took a short break to take her son and his schoolmates back to school. Faine had borrowed her digital camera so he could photograph his and his friends' artwork during class. He excitedly showed his mother the photos he had taken. Faine's mother shared a story about one of Faine's art projects that sold at an art auction fundraiser. He was sent a check for half the value of the sale. The other half went back to the studio. Faine was so proud he wanted to frame the check, but his mother compromised by photocopying the check for him.

The list of Faine's capabilities continued to unfold during observations at special school. For example, at senior prize giving he was awarded for his leadership in the school's kapa haka cultural group. As part of the school's literacy focus, he printed and bound a book he wrote and illustrated with the support of his teachers. Crafts he had made throughout the year as part of a business enterprise group were proudly offered for sale at a market day in the local shopping mall. Faine did not come to school that day to sell his artwork. It was said that there were family issues at home.

Two of the most defining moments observed of Faine's school success were as stereotypical as any other student's transition - the school ball (prom) and graduation. The ball was a joint effort between two special schools, and was held at the community satellite classroom at Faine's school. Overall, the ball had a pleasant, happy vibe. Everyone was well dressed. Four tables were filled with food, mostly prepared by students or brought in by family as a shared plate. The plentiful amount of food at the ball served as a metaphoric demonstration of the abundance of collective love for the schools and one another. Students supported one another. For example, those in and out of wheelchairs danced together. Students with verbal abilities sang karaoke, yet held the microphone for participation of those without verbal abilities. The most noticeable thing was an absence; the absence of antisocial behaviors from any of the students in attendance.

Faine was dressed up as his favorite singer. He had fake tattoos on his hands and neck. During the ball, he performed with his band. The school principal even joined the band for the evening. Soon after, the king and queen of the ball were announced. The queen was a young woman in a wheelchair dressed in an elegant Indian sari. Faine won king of the ball. He was so hot from all his singing and dancing that the sweat could almost be mistaken for tears of joy. There was, however, no mistaking his beaming, proud smile (photograph collected, in-school phase).

Later in the week was graduation, which was again held at the school. Families and guests of the school were asked to wait outside so they could be formally welcomed through a powhiri, a Māori welcoming ceremony to greet visitors. The powhiri was led by Faine's mother and members of his whānau family. In between graduation speeches from the school community, principal, and teachers, waiata or Māori language songs, were sung by most in attendance. The school principal introduced the graduation ceremony, stating to the students "we have learned far more from you than you've ever learned from us" (Quote transcript, in-school phase). Each graduate was introduced through a photographic slide show. Family photos were set alongside photos collected during the graduate's time at school, and each slideshow was set to preferred music. Teachers then shared more specific comments about their graduates. The principal gave each a gift, mostly Māori carvings in greenstone.

Faine was the last graduate presentation. He sobbed, crying throughout his whole slideshow. His family cried, too. His family again sang a waiata for him in Māori. Then the school's cultural group led a haka (a traditional, ancestral, postured, rhythmic group dance) in his honor. In this final moment, it was clear how integral Faine and his family had become to the school. Faine's contribution to the school had almost been larger than life and he would be sincerely missed.

Timetable As part of a photographic adapted interview, Faine was asked to demonstrate features of his classroom that were important to him. Of the range of photos collected and described, Faine took one of his classroom timetable. There was one timetable for the whole class, and it listed activities with classmates' pictures associated with who would be participating in each activity. Faine's comments about the photo were literal and straightforward:

Sarah: What's this next one?

Faine: Morning circle, [work experience at the department store], gym, and bocce.

Sarah: Is this your class timetable?

Faine: Yeah, class timetable and what we are doing. Like lunch then ...

Sarah: That's how you know what you're doing for the day. (Interview transcript, Faine, in-school phase)

Faine demonstrated with this quote that he understood the component elements that made up his classroom timetable. The use of picture communication symbols (PCS) supplemented the text and enabled him to "read" the information. Furthermore, he could distinguish between his own daily activities and those of his peers by way of student photographs. In a photographic interview, Faine conveyed that timetables held personal relevance. Notably, he raised the priority of this topic of timetables himself.

SECTION 2: POST-SCHOOL: COMMUNITY DAY PROGRAM

While still in school, Faine made a few visits to the community participation day service he was to attend after he left school. He was only able to go a few times due to scheduling conflicts between the school and the day service. He was supported by a teacher aide at his special school who described,

I do have a few concerns. They take a long time to set up and organize staffing. Mind you, they don't have Faine in the first session, he's there for the second session. Faine and peers arrive [to the day service] and they have lunch, and it takes them a while to set up the afternoon activities. Faine runs out of time for a thorough visit because his school day then finishes. (Faine's two teachers interview transcript, in-school phase)

Faine's stress levels began to rise the more he visited the post-school day service. His mother commented this resulted in an increase in Faine's antisocial behaviors at home. These behaviors were not observed at school, but then some days Faine would mysteriously be away from school. Faine's mother commented that he associated his fears about the new day program with not wanting to go to school at all. His mother raised the issue of rising stress levels in an interview,

Faine's mother: He's pretty anxious at the moment. I'm pretty anxious at the moment. It's like the unknown, really. I think we're going to hit a few behaviors, maybe.
Sarah: What do his behaviors look like? Anxiety?
Faine's mother: Yeah. He hasn't had any violent episodes, but occasionally he will, and you know it's a big overload, so I just stop everything. And wait for him to get back on track. And he's teary for a few days.
Sarah: Oh, because he was absent the other day, when I was supposed to see him.

Faine's mother: He turned into this really horrible child.

Sarah: I couldn't imagine!

Faine's mother: Verbal like a wolverine. And physical and everything. And you point your finger and then he dumps it all on the ground. And it's always been focused at me. But his brother is the one to be stern with him, to say that's enough, and go to bed. Or go to your room or something. And then the next day he just feels absolutely horrified at what he's done. So then we have two to three days of feeling like, oh my g-d why did I do that? I've hurt feelings and upset people. He gets anxious over that too.

Sarah: He's so sensitive, that's what I've found.

Faine's mother: So we just go through that process.

Sarah: He doesn't do that at school, does he? Just for you?

Faine's mother: Ah, no, he stopped doing any of that when we went to special school. He was really, really bad up until then. My main focus was for him to get on with people and social skills, and the rest I didn't care about. That's what we needed to work on. And he's come a long way. (Faine's mother, interview transcript, in-school phase)

Faine's community day service was located in an industrial park. A mechanic and boat supply warehouse were on either side of the day service's building. During the first visit, Faine was observed lying on the couch with his shoes off, feet up, and an icepack on his forehead. He complained of heat stroke after a walk outside. The day was sunny, though cool in comparison to the previous days of high humidity.

In conversation, he was initially quiet and unenthusiastic but then perked up when he began to reminisce about special school. He had been invited back to school to attend his former classmate's 21st birthday. At that moment, one of his former classmates walked past, who was non-verbal, and communicated by jumping and making noises like, "ha!" Faine's attitude soured as he noted that he couldn't remember this young adult's name. Though he didn't state it directly, it was apparent that most of Faine's potential peers at the day service were similar to this former classmate. They used non-verbal or semi-verbal restricted communication. Throughout the observation, whenever Faine spoke about special school, he was happy. When his current life at the day service was mentioned, his attitude dulled.

In an interview with the day program's coordinator, she described Faine's progress as seeming small, but improvements were noticeable and goals achievable when set to his pace. She gave examples like taking initiative to pour himself a drink of water. Faine had begun an adapted sailing activity the previous week and begrudgingly approached sailing with his hoody on, a gesture that indicated his feeling unsure. By the end of the experience, Faine was reported to be overjoyed by learning a new skill and overcoming his fear of a new activity. Yet, during the next fieldwork observation to visit the sailing site, Faine did not show up. With no responses to phone or written messages, the following email arrived a week later,

> Hi Sarah,
> It has been a sad time for our extended family.
> It has not been a very smooth transition for Faine from special school and we have all had a lot of emotional challenges and hurdles to work through. [Associate Principal] and our special school whānau have given so much, helped bring out the best qualities in Faine, and always made him part of the decisions and choices he needed to make to take his life on a pathway that made him happy and that was good for him.
> Challenge, laughter, independence, learning, and love was what Faine received and gave every day. Unfortunately, he is missing these very important things during this transition and is finding it very hard. It is hard when all your child wants is to be included when making choices in his daily activities and all he wants is to have a day when his life is filled with so much laughter that your sides hurt and you are still smiling hours after. We will continue to keep striving for those things. Thank you for everything. We will see each other again soon.Faine & his mother. (Email transcript, post-school phase)

It transpired that Faine had gone with his family to a tangi, a ceremonial Māori funeral, which typically lasts about a week. Despite trying to get in touch, the research ended abruptly without seeing Faine or his mother again.

Timetable In an observation during the post-school phase, a timetable was on the wall of the day service above where Faine was sitting. The observation was described in field notes,

> When asked about the timetable pinned to the wall, Faine says he can't read it and suggests the one at special school was better. The one at the day service was written in small, handwritten lettering for the whole week (rather than daily as it was at his special school) and used no picture symbols. When

asked what activity is coming up after lunch, Faine offers a few suggestions, but none prove to be correct. (Field notes, post-school phase)

In the post-school phase of the community day service, Faine appeared lost. The timetable used in the community day service was likely most useful to the staff as a way to organize what was going on, where, and when. While in school Faine had demonstrated the capabilities to track the progression of his day, as well as the ability to situate his day in relation to the activities of his peers. The special school afforded him access to a timetable that was meaningful to him. These skills were lost in the transition process between in-school and post-school.

Section 3: Transition

The progression of Faine's transition turned from unexpected and resounding positivity, akin to the discovery and successful use of his school's symbol timetable, to challenges post-school, analogous to the hand-written weekly timetable that Faine could not read nor understand. Might it have been that in transition, his brief and successful time at special school was too good to replace? Or maybe Faine and his mother simply need more time to work through Faine's significant life challenges? Such questions may be moot. By the end of fieldwork, it was unclear whether Faine would continue post-school community services. His whānau family's answer to the stresses of transition appeared to be to return Faine, once again, into their protection. This may have been his whānau's way of coping with Faine's reaction to his post-school program.

ANZ Conclusion

The three case narratives from ANZ revealed three transition realities. For Haku, transition appeared successful, drawing on consistent supports and familiar artifacts such as his timetable in the in-school and post-school contexts. In contrast, Cobain experienced challenges in both environments, akin to how timetables (or ideas for timetables) existed, but were never fully utilized. Finally, Faine moved from strength to post-school distress. The timetable he used successfully in school was discontinued in the post-school context making his new schedule inaccessible. Timetables were one useful way to consider the consistency or the degree to which each young man experienced a successful transition. Beyond the success or quality of the transition outcome, timetables also enabled consideration of how each young man eventuated to each point of success or struggle.

The elements that constituted a timetable, the activities and priorities set within them, conveyed vital elements of personal priority. Transportation, cooking, and kapa haka cultural group, for example, were important activities, and show how an appropriately implemented timetable could scaffold dignified daily engagement. Timetables were personalized. They included information such as how long it was appropriate to expect each young man to be engaged in particular activities, or how often activities typically occurred. In turn, timetables also provided a communicative element by enabling each young man's ability to convey, share, assess, and structure their understanding of their transition, as well as the transitions of their peers.

United States

The time point has now shifted. This section depicts the years spanning the Covid-19 pandemic and regionally specific lockdowns. A composite narrative is presented of a young adult named El.

Since the El's case is an amalgamation of the experiences of many young adults with disabilities, only one narrative represents USA. Of note, there was no direct inquiry specifically about post-school transition during the American Voices Project (AVP) interviews. Therefore, transition was reflected through the liminal progression from in-school to post-school. Interview probes determined by the AVP form the subheadings within the narrative. Almost the entire narrative was written in direct quotes woven together from multiple interview transcripts. Minimal edits were made to enhance the flow and readability in compiling the composite case.

The presentation of the ANZ narratives were joined together through a tangible anchor of a timetable. Yet, no such calendar or organizer was specifically discussed within the AVP transcripts in USA. The closest resemblance depicted within El's case was a waitlist. The young adults in ANZ had the opportunity, though sometimes inconsistently, to contribute to and monitor their schedules. Life events for El in USA were chaotic and unstable, oftentimes too unpredictable for such organization. Instead, what El most regularly experienced both in school and out was the passivity of having to wait. While this was consistently experienced throughout El's composite narrative, it was not used as any sort of assessment of the "success" of El's transition. Rather, a narrative was constructed of important life markers during a time of considerable instability.

El

My name is El. I am living in the suburbs of Southwestern USA. I am Hispanic and of mixed race, unemployed, with no kids, and am single. I graduated high school and am politically independent.

I've lived everywhere, coast to coast. My mom made a lot of bad decisions when I was growing up, so we moved around a lot. Never stayed in the same place for over a year. We ended up on the streets sometimes. Sometimes in shelters to get out of the rain. I don't need much, except to get out of the rain.

I know that I have been treated differently all of my life because of my mixed race. I have grown up with it, so I have gotten used to it and it doesn't bother me. My grandmother rolled her Rs so much when reading us bedtime stories in English—it made the kids laugh! But being treated differently bothers my mother. Like when she goes shopping and gets followed around in the store. She wasn't treated the same way as her workmates at her job. Me, I just always dealt with it. People don't like to hear this, but it's very racist out there. I am half Mexican, but have white-looking skin, so I was bullied a lot. Jumped by three kids when I was at school. They didn't see me as Mexican, so it's constant racism.

My disabilities are related to my health, mental and physical. I was diagnosed with schizophrenia. I was diagnosed with schizophrenia because I was really into anime and then I started being able to see and hear the characters. I was 13 when I was diagnosed, and couldn't find a doctor to get a second opinion. I didn't like therapy, but now I realize that I need it. Right now, I sleep for about 12 hours a night, but sometimes I sleep only two hours. That's when I have stress and anxiety. When I can't sleep, my leg shakes. I have to hold my legs down. My heart races, and it keeps me up. I've tried CBD (cannabidiol cannabis), pills, chakra necklaces, stones, nothing helps my stress.

People stress me out because they think that I am going to cause myself a heart attack. They say I should rest and relax. It's stressful sometimes. I get tired and out of breath helping my sister because she needs care for everything. My older sister got in a car wreck six years ago and she became paralyzed. We have different mindsets now. She pushed me to have higher expectations.

There are lots of emotions that come up with a physical disability, like my heart condition and my back injury. I also have depression. Not the suicidal kind, but I always feel alone. I don't have many friends, really don't have anyone outside of my family. So, I started talking to myself. Just for company. I stay in my pajamas, I don't get dressed for anything. I can't work because I can't stand for long periods of time. If I do my shopping, after standing in long lines, I am done for the day. My whole body hurts. Mentally I'm not in the place I want to be right now because of my health, but spiritually I'm in a good place. And I still have my optimism.

COMMUNITY SETTINGS

Living away from the city, there isn't too much to do. My mom is from Mexico and there are no Hispanics in this suburban town; very little diversity. If we want anything related to our culture, we have to go 45 minutes away to the capital city, like for the types of food we need.

In the neighborhoods we used to live in there was a lot of criminal stuff. Break-ins to the apartments, people with guns, people that get drunk and are firing guns. There's a lot of bad stuff that happened there. My brother joined a gang. The first time I was shot at I was age 11. I was living on and off the streets by the age of 12. I've had a gun to my face so many times it's hilarious.

The apartments we lived in were a bit of trash. We lived under Housing and Urban Development (HUD). They're low-income apartments. We were crammed into a small space, and gang life, such as drugs started coming into the town. So, we moved again to strike the right balance of cultural diversity, a perfect mix where there are resources and people who spoke Spanish. But then rents started to rise.

What is important to me now is life outside the city. I can see mountains. Hear birds. There are only three stores and they're each a mile away. This aspect of my town is paradise. This is happiness. The neighbors in my neighborhood are pretty good, and good to me. Sometimes they do things like set off fireworks in the middle of April. And there's crime and stuff like that, but to me, nothing is too serious, nothing too extreme.

FAMILY AND IDENTITY

We are a large family. Mom is one of five kids. My dad was one of four. I had a crazy childhood. I was raised poor. I was not shielded from anything, every day it was like one thing after another. It was a kind of I raised myself sort of standard. It was pretty okay. I learned a lot of things and they made me mature fast.

My parents were alcoholics. That stretched our budget even tighter. I thought they just drank a lot. I didn't see a lot of beatings. But sometimes. I thought a lot of their fighting was because of me coming out. After my parents divorced, my mom had a new partner. This man was incredibly abusive to me, and I think to her at a time. My childhood was very fraught with physical abuse. I became really shy, because if I would speak, my mother's partner would yell. A lot of my treatment in therapy comes back to the fact that I really needed my mother as a kid, and she wasn't there. She wasn't there to keep me safe.

And then, when I'd go into my father's house, I'd experience the trauma of neglect and emotional distance. That was really hard for me. In my teen years, I struggled a lot with depression, which is still an ongoing struggle, but as a younger person, I didn't have any tools or resources to really deal with that in the way that I needed to.

We tried to live the American dream as we considered it, but we were on a tight budget growing up. We would get donations like shoes from the church. The church was a big part of our lives. We lived off food stamps and housing subsidies. Mom worried about money all the time. My clothes didn't fit. We had to get away from mom's partner, so we moved with no money. Some people would say who cares about that family because they're undocumented. It seemed like we were a bag of meat to them. Child Protective Services (CPS), they knew who we were. At age 4 or 5 my mom got all of us kids diagnosed at the psychiatrist, so we could receive disability welfare payouts. She was living off our checks.

I was tired of wearing shoes with my toes curled up because they didn't fit. I was tired of being hungry. So, I got a fake ID that said I was 18 when I was 13 and started working. I worked in a movie theater as a janitor. When I actually turned 18, I finally confronted my mom about using the kids' disability welfare payouts. We went down to the Social Security office, and they gave me my Social Security card and confirmed that the payments were for me. When we left, my mom told me never to ask her for anything ever again. She said, don't come, don't ask me for anything. I will never ever, ever buy you anything. That money helped me have a life, get a place to live, work somewhere, get up, stay with people where they were actually like, you need to pay rent. I live a good life off this money. I have food, a room, clean clothes.

Growing up, I made my family's life a lot harder because of coming out about my sexual orientation. Who I was. I think that made my parents end their marriage. I first came out to my aunt. She was drunk when I told her, and we kept it as our secret for a while. Then, she got drunk at Thanksgiving and told everyone about our secret. Mom thought she was lying, but why would I continue a lie? That year was the worst of my life. My mom got violent, broke doors, and my parents' marriage unraveled. She thought it was because I went to juvenile detention for a few months, and was maybe raped. But nothing like that happened to me there. I've heard stories like that from other people, but it wasn't my experience. I was so stressed when I came out that I used to drink a lot. I'd come home drunk. I dated someone who was 15 years older than me. They would buy me alcohol and get me into nightclubs. Due to all the drama, I almost didn't finish school.

I have pursued the coming out process on my own over the last five years. I think a lot of us experience different traumas in our lives, or think that's what we are experiencing at a younger age. But when you are young, things feel more exploratory or more just sort of curious. I experienced a lot of shame, especially from my parents, which I think ultimately comes from their fear and uncertainty around a healthy exploration of gender.

In-school

In high school, by the way I dressed, I got bullied. People said I looked gay. I got called fat, because of the medication I was taking for my mental health made me gain weight. I spent most of my time crying in my guidance counselor's office. I don't want to remember those times. They still haunt me. I was literally the only white complexion student in a school filled with brown and black kids, so that was not an easy task. Every time people would try to mess with me, I'd stand up for myself, of course, but then I'd be the one getting kicked out of school every time. There were too many kids at my urban school, so we never had direct information about how to get help. I was always misinformed—not enough communication with teachers happening.

Another problem with my high school was the schools I went to, you had to walk through metal detectors to get in. They had onsite police guards. Police, actual city police. It just sucks when you go to school and then they have something called random searches. They just walk into a classroom. Tell you to come outside, bring all of your stuff and they will literally take everything out of your backpack. They'll dump it all on the floor, making sure you have nothing on you. This is what I come to school for? To be treated like a fucking criminal? That was my school experience.

I had learning disabilities. My mom saw that I was having trouble in the urban schools, and she knew my cousins in the rural area were happy at school, so it worked out when we moved that I was successful there. Surprisingly, I received a better education in the rural areas. At my rural school, teachers were really part of student's lives. We were actually starting to live a life that we deserved as children.

I was lucky to have diversity in my rural school, but some of my younger siblings weren't as lucky. They actually dropped out and went to an alternative school to get away from some of the rude things they experienced. They had to endure a lot. Neighbors threw dog shit at the house. School was crushing their spirit.

The only reason why I went to school, to be honest, is because my dad passed away when I was in high school, so I was getting survivor benefits for attending school. It was kind of like getting paid to go to school. My family needed so much help that it was hard to focus on my studies. For example, mom used us kids as translators, so we'd miss a lot of school. School staff would come to the house to take us to school because we were missing too much.

After high school, I enrolled in college, but didn't feel like I was learning anything. I switched to a tech school, and felt like I actually learned more there.

POST-SCHOOL LIFE

I keep to the same daily routines. Just get up, try to shake off the back pain, feed the cats, watch TV, and that's it. I don't work, so I don't get out much. The only people that come around might be someone from my family. I don't have a vehicle, so I walk, mostly to the dollar store nearby. Walk and take the bus. The main place that I go in the community is to the pool with my mom on her days off work.

Sometimes I catch myself getting bored. I want a job to do something other than be bored. I'm thinking about volunteering. My aunt helps protect pit bulls. I might help her. I love pit bulls, I did my senior project in high school on their history and abuse.

I also love drawing. It's the only way I put up with the boredom. It helps me. It's a stress relief. But depression still comes and goes. Just like my ability to draw. Sometimes it comes, a talent, it comes, and it goes.

I'm pretty much stuck at home for the most part, not able to really do a whole lot apart from physical therapy on Thursday. After physical therapy, I'm able to feel almost normal again, walk around, and do something I need to do on a Friday, like get a haircut or cleaning and organizing the house.

Growing up I wanted to be the best example I can for my siblings. Whatever I do my siblings reflect. I have two brothers, one is in prison for murder. The other is a real dumbass. They took his kids off him. I went to go and try to sort him out. I don't care what he did, he's my brother. I did what I could to sort out my family. Get them on good footing, build their life back up.

Then, I got a call from my granny and that set everything into motion. I relocated to a different part of the country motivated by my grandma being sick. She was living in my stepfather's basement, but he has a history of being abusive. So, I found a place and moved her in with me. I looked after her end-of-life care.

Employment Growing up my father focused on work, and our relationship to work was really important to him, which is messing up my life now. In the past, I had a job working at a movie theater. And that was my first job in my whole entire life. I have never ever, ever had a job. Till this day, I still receive Social Security income. I receive disability income. I would give it up to start my life and my job. I tell myself this every day.

I didn't get paid enough to keep going at that movie theater job. $10 an hour, it should have been like $13. I get emotional really easy. I argued with my boss about my pay, and then I went into the bathroom and cried. So I left the job. I kinda regret leaving, because I thought that with that job my life was going to change. I was going to get friends, share phone numbers, and send texts. I cried a lot the next week because none of that happened.

I worked for a little while recently as a self-employed landscaper, a job my father did. But then I got a back injury. I won't go back to working in landscaping anyway because of the workers' rights issues I saw while working there. Like co-workers from Guatemala here on a work visa welding for $4 an hour - this is completely unacceptable. Another of my co-workers got fired right before I left because she had really bad PTSD [post-traumatic stress disorder] and they thought she was crazy because she was willing to speak up. I want to move on, and I really want a job so I can get more of my own stuff with my own money. For extra money, I sometimes use a cash app or sell plasma.

My main future focus is to have stable money. To be able to go out a buy a phone if I need one. My whole life money stability has been an issue. Money doesn't fix everything, but it would help. It's silly, I know, but I would just love that. I could start somewhere.

Programs and services I just moved, and I realize that I need to find a therapist. My health insurance switched when moving. I am on a waiting list for a program to help me. All the moving makes me confused sometimes. The roadblock to my success is waitlists for programs.

I need to have a medical procedure but I can't find someone to drive me from the appointment, so I need to wait for my mom to visit and stay awhile. The type of physical therapy that I need isn't covered by insurance. So, it's all out of pocket for me. I can only afford once a week and I'm barely doing that. There have been occasions where I might not be able to afford therapy and I will skip a week or two. It just gets real bad if I'm not able to do it, but unfortunately that's all I'm able to afford right now. If I could have therapy done twice a week I'd pretty much be feeling normal 24/7, then I'd be off disability and able to work again. They are so restrictive about it, so it won't happen unfortunately.

Drugs I don't drink or smoke because I'm on lots of prescribed medications and I don't want bad complications. I don't take any pills unless they are prescribed to me. I hate taking pills. Even with the prescribed ones I have to be careful not to get too addicted. Especially the ones for pain. Sometimes I only take half of what they tell me to so that I don't get addicted to it. I used to have a drinking problem. Now I drink only very little. I sometimes smoke weed and take CBD for pain management.

Relationships I've had relationships before. I dated someone who was 29 when I was 14. I didn't tell my age. I looked older. By being in this relationship, I could get into clubs and buy alcohol. My parents wondered why I was coming home drunk. I kept this relationship a secret. Another person I dated struggled with severe post-traumatic stress disorder (PTSD). There was a lot of time spent on navigating health and mental health.

My commitment now is to stand on my own before I have a committed relationship. I've seen other people lose their freedom in relationships. I can be my own person. I don't like public displays of affection anyway, people are too judgmental.

Police I never counted on law enforcement growing up. You could call them, but they'd never show up. I had to keep a low profile from the police because I was the only white-looking person in the city. If someone described a white person for a crime, I'd be accused for everything.

When I was 18, I was arrested for panhandling. I was put in a cell with others coming in and out all night. I was allowed to go on my merry way the next day, it didn't amount to anything. But what I shared in common with all the other folks coming through is that the police didn't care about any of us. I saw one woman have menstrual bleeding all over her white dress. I saw another go into diabetic shock, faint, then crack her head on the toilet. I saw another person coming down off of a crack addiction. All these people who were all having different experiences, but we were all in the same place together, but the thing that we all shared is that the police didn't give a fuck. It didn't matter what experiences were happening, they didn't care. It didn't matter if it was a medical emergency, or a hygiene issue, or a public health thing. It didn't matter to them.

Politics and voting If I vote for someone, my priority is on their support of independency. My political view is that lawmakers should serve for a few years, but then need to step out of the role so that they can live under the laws they created. If you're going to be in leadership, walk a mile in someone else's shoes. Learn what it's like to be someone other than yourself. Walk a mile, because it's easy to say I know what your problem is. It really is that you don't know until you've been there.

I vote. I do a lot of research before I go to vote on the day. Everyone should. Most of my information comes from Fox News. I get a lot of my information from them, at the same time, I actually go online at do some more research. No matter the results of voting, I am going to still be happy. I just don't have that much energy for politics. I don't have enough energy to get all my information right.

The thing I care about mostly is the people's right to live their lives, the freedom of speech. Freedom, the thing that makes this country. The thing that makes everybody in this world wanting to come here. I strongly believe we live in the greatest nation ever built. Our homeless live better than most people in the world. I'm a living example of that.

Disability Justice isn't just about being good to people with disabilities and making sure somebody in a wheelchair can fit through a door. It's the deeper work of relating to people, understanding people, and building culture and context together. It's not a question about whether we have sign language (ASL) at our trainings. That's just a part of it.

Hopes and dreams during pandemic times I believe there has been a collective reckoning about how we live in the world. We take care of each other. During the pandemic, if I am heading to the store, I'll ask my neighbors if they need anything. We share with each other, even if we have nothing. People who are most disproportionately affected by the pandemic are the people who are able to care for each other the best.

I didn't change anything in my life due to Covid. I figure if I survived my bullshit childhood life then I can survive anything. At the start of the pandemic, I had to go two months without physical therapy. That was bad, I had to rely only on pain medications - pills, patches, and creams. The only times when I feel close to normal is after therapy. I always have to be careful what I do with how my body is going to react to any activity. There have been times where I try to be more active, but the next day, oh man, I'll end up in bed for days after.

Where there were Covid impacts, they were mostly about a young member of my family who turned 5 at the time. It wasn't fun to home school a child who was just starting school. I was lucky cause I had time since I was on a disability benefit, and my financials didn't change. The other impact was the health of my sister because she only uses 60% capacity of her lungs after her accident, so we need to be very careful around her. Mostly it's just hard to only socialize with people online or on the phone. I prefer to stay off social media as much as possible because it makes life more stressful, and I don't really need to use it. If I need to get in touch with someone, I can call them directly.

In the future, I hope to be different from where I am now. Hopefully, I have a successful career in something I enjoy, whether it's something to do with art, or helping the community, like I said, with the pit bulls, helping them out. I'm not really a people person, but I love animals, and I want to help them. I want to eventually get my license. I want to do something more with my life than just sleep and not do anything. I wake up, and I'm like, this is not the life I want to be living. I want to change it.

Transition commentary El is waiting for life to change. Returning to the reoccurring theme of waitlists, El waited while in school for teachers' attention within a crowded school, and waited for educational support that was in short supply due to lack of funding. These waits became so extreme, the family moved to a new part of the country to attend school in a rural area with smaller student populations. Due to El's transience, post-school life typically involved being placed on waitlists for services, such as mental health counseling and support groups, or access to medical treatments such as specific physical therapies. El's narrative does not include any sort of positive or negative assessment of the "success" of transition. Rather, a narrative is constructed of pivotal life experiences that led up to and then occurred following, the exit from school. All occurred during a time of significant instability. El describes an optimism for the future but takes almost no actions to make positive changes for the future. Instead, El waits.

Chapter Conclusion

In this chapter, four narrative cases were presented between the countries of ANZ and USA. The first three cases in ANZ were joined together by a symbolic representation of the timetable, whereas the final narrative from USA was metaphorically depicted through a waitlist. Cases from ANZ occurred five years before the pandemic, and the USA case occurred directly during Covid-19-associated lockdowns. Each case developed by adhering to the theoretical commitments of capability in that every young adult had a story to tell that contributes valuable knowledge to the subject of post-school transition. Until this point, each case was presented free from theoretical commentary. The focus of the next chapter is to apply capability theory to improve the opportunity for a transition with dignity.

References

Bengtsson, M. (2016). How to plan and perform a qualitative study using content analysis. *Nursing Plus Open, 2,* 8–14. https://doi.org/10.1016/j.npls.2016.01.001

Hart, S. M., Hill, M. F., & Gaffney, J. S. (2021). Timetabling a transition with dignity: Perspectives of young adults with significant support needs. *Journal of Intellectual and Developmental Disability, 46*(3), 227–238. https://doi.org/10.3109/13668250.2021.1885973

Johnston, O., Wildy, H., & Shand, J. (2023). Student voices that resonate: Constructing composite narratives that represent students' classroom experiences. *Qualitative Research, 23*(1), 108–124. https://doi.org/10.1177/14687941211016158

CHAPTER 6

Transition with Dignity

Abstract This chapter opens with a possibility-based discussion whereby each of the young adults' transitions is reconsidered through the lens of the capability approach. Description of key themes shared between the cases include: (a) dignity of risk, or the right to make one's own decisions despite reasonable hazards, and (b) trailing, or exploring more inclusive opportunities that align with an individual's capability set. Together, addressing dignity in post-school transition practices can lead to a genuine opportunity for all.

Keywords Adapted preferences • Dignity • Dignity of risk • Metaphor • Trialing

> Just by being human, all are of equal dignity and worth, no matter where they are situated in society, and the primary source of this worth is a power of moral choice within them, a power that consists in the ability to plan a life in accordance with one's own evaluation of ends (Nussbaum, 2006, p. 57).

POSSIBILITY OVER PROBLEMS

Dignity, the term used in the book title, signals theoretical commitments of an aspirational purpose. Even when dignity was not routinely experienced within the transitions depicted, this chapter demonstrates ways that dignity remains a viable opportunity for future transitions. To achieve this, problems associated with transition should not be ignored, yet cannot overshadow the considerations for more positive results. Essentially, a focus on possibility over problems (Gaffney, 2013).

Adapted preferences With an already problematic stereotype of post-school transition, there is another issue that further compounds the challenges. Nussbaum and other moral philosophers refer to a phenomenon called adapted preferences (Nussbaum, 2011). Namely, that certain conditions are made more problematic because we expect or collude in making them be so, such that longstanding circumstances overtime become no longer questioned. The classic example of adapted preferences comes from the Aesop fable of sour grapes. Since a bunch of grapes was too high for the fox to reach, he decided that they were likely unripe and sour, therefore undesirable and not worth trying for. With a complicated historical legacy, it becomes reasonable to question how much of the disability experience, and transition more specifically, has become soured by adapted preferences.

Multiple examples of adaptive preferences can be found within the young adults' transitions. Some of the transition support networks, such as parents and families, were so adjusted to transition being associated with hardship, that they didn't question these circumstances. They may have even found adversity preferably predictable, or relatable to the transitions they previously heard about from others in the disability community. Adapted preferences thus impacted methodological decisions not to survey participants for well-being, because those involved with transition may have professed satisfaction with unjust conditions. They had adjusted their expectations.

As the prior chapters have asserted, active citizenship of individuals with significant disabilities following school depends as much upon in-school procedures and systems as it does the inclusivity of society itself. Adaptative preferences have obscured certain long-held prejudices that impact social structures and community engagement. The intentional methodological decision to put the two countries of ANZ and USA alongside facilitates the ability to consider the topic of transition from "upside down." The distinct socio-political and philosophical foundations of disability rights in each country have led to qualitatively different expectations and transition experiences. Rather than hardships being presented to dissect the problems of transition, they were shared for problems to make way for the opportunity to consider transition in new ways.

We now return to Haku, Cobain, Faine, and El. Trying to examine beyond the challenges involved in their transitions, the possibilities of transition are framed through capability metaphors assigned to each case. The central underlying assumption in each metaphor was that everyone, regardless of disability status, has the capability to contribute to both their transition and to research on this topic. Each symbolic metaphor is discussed in direction connection with the personal capabilities demonstrated during post-school transition.

Capability Metaphors

ANZ

Haku A public transportation map (Fig. 6.1) serves as Haku's transition symbol. The map represents the freedoms and opportunities that open up when one is capable of using route planning maps and public transportation timetables. In urban ANZ, school students do not commonly have access to school bus transportation to and from school. In primary (elementary)

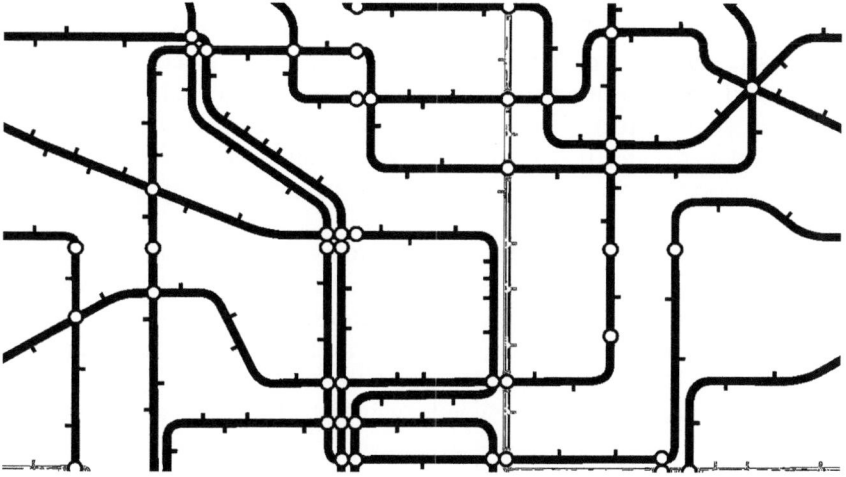

Fig. 6.1 Haku's transition metaphor: Transit map

school years, students typically walk or are driven to school by their parents. In secondary school years, students may walk, bike, or use public transportation. This is not the case for students attending special school as these students have taxi transportation funded to and from school each day.

Locations that Haku was known to go throughout fieldwork were geo-located. When reliant upon external transportation supports, such as a taxi and his mother, he went to places in an approximately 16-kilometer (10-mile) radius from his home. Even though Haku's polytechnic program was for students with disability, he and his peers were expected to arrange their campus transportation. Furthermore, Haku continued to go from work experience to course once per week. Due to the aforementioned transportation support during his school years, Haku never had the need or opportunity to use public transportation. Despite this, Haku's transition team supported him in learning to use a very complicated urban public transportation system. Strikingly, not only did Haku learn to use transportation to get himself to and from his course and work, but he also began using transportation for leisure. During post-school fieldwork, Haku was known to have explored on his own initiative, places such as the beach, the shopping mall, and new suburbs he had never been to before. From these excursions, his travel expanded to an approximately 42-kilometer (26-mile) radius from his home.

Haku's symbol of a transportation map represents the differences between the taxi, with a predetermined route that was not necessarily set by Haku, and the freedom public transportation afforded him. In this symbol, Haku's transition success can be understood not solely in terms of personal achievement (i.e., increase of 26-kilometer/16-mile distance) but in opportunities that opened up to him after having learned to use public transportation. Haku had autonomy over his community access.

Capability discussion Through in-school to post-school transition, Haku moved from strength to strength. He demonstrated personal capabilities almost no one could ignore. Success was represented by the pictures on the walls of his in-school classroom, such as his skills at his workplace, and continued through his lessons at polytechnic. In imagining Haku's future, one might first reflect on his past to wonder why he had attended a special school in the first place. How might his experiences have been different were he to have transitioned from a mainstream school? Might he, for example, have been able to break out of disability-specific contexts as he had demonstrated in the examples of transportation and work experience? Maybe he could have enrolled at a polytechnic in a mainstream program, instead of a course only for students with disability? Given what was gleaned from the interview with Haku's polytechnic instructor, it may unfortunately be predicted that his transition outcome would have ended up the same despite his educational placement during his in-school years. Procedural barriers, such as graduation certificate standards and post-secondary education entry criteria continue to restrict educational options for students with disabilities.

In concluding Haku's narrative, recall how many of his accomplishments were achieved on his own initiative. For example, no one told Haku to use transportation for leisure. In the same manner, Haku led his transition team to facilitate his continued work experience during his tertiary education. Furthermore, it was only by chance, not by design, that the format of timetable diaries between in-school and post-school contexts was similar. A concluding question is how much of Haku's transition was by luck, chance, or most strikingly, through his personal skills, interest, and determination, rather than strategically planned for by his transition team?

Cobain Some additional background information is first provided about the roundabout manner in which Cobain's transition was funded to enable intensive or one-to-one staffing for his post-school activities. Cobain and his family chose an individualized program following school, rather than, for example, a day service care program. The central activity of his individualized program was therapeutic horseback riding, an expensive activity. Stretching disability support funding as far as it could go, the decision was made for him to receive eight hours of one-to-one support per week. Then, out of what would typically be a ten-hour week of support, a supplemental activity fee was provided by the residential care service to pay for the costs associated with the horse riding. Transportation to and from horse riding counted as part of the eight total hours. Eight hours were then stretched further when Cobain shared staff with other housemates and those in the residential service, which occurred during the adapted art lesson described in the prior chapter.

(Un)locked doors signified Cobain's transition. As portrayed in the details of his narrative, Cobain's transition involved emotions and stress for his transition team. Specifically, his mother. Cobain spent great lengths of time away from the tension, preferring quieter spaces. Like exit doors. In the left-hand side of Fig. 6.2 (image intentionally blurred for anonymity),

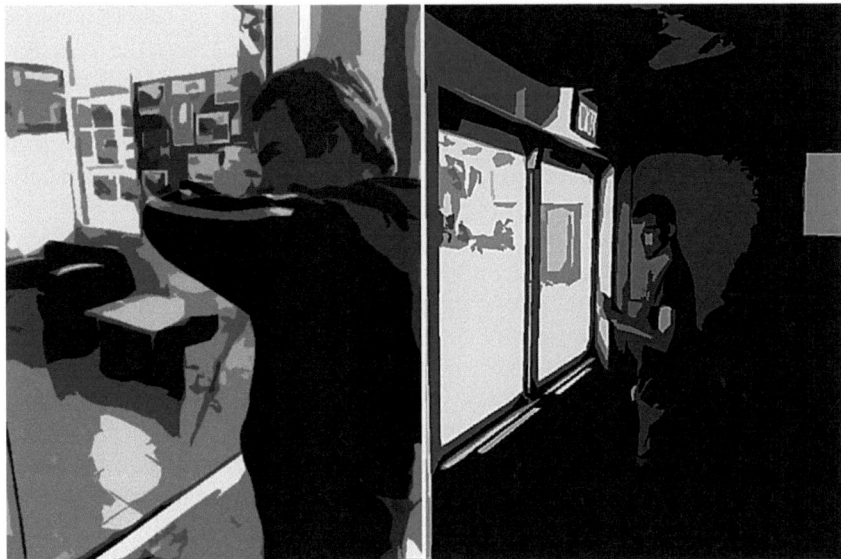

Fig. 6.2 Cobain's transition metaphor: (Un)locked doors

a photo taken at his special school, the main doors were made of rein-
forced glass. He enjoyed standing by the doors to watch bursts of sunlight
and reflections that appealed to him, given his visual impairment. This was
one of his spaces of calm much like the olive grove shown during an initial
observation. The time spent at the school doors far exceeded observations
of engagement in scheduled curriculum, with classmates, or participation
in class activities. Stories were shared amongst school staff members about
times when a new person, such as a relief (substitute) staff member, would
join the class. Cobain would demonstrate his knowledge of the door's
purpose when he would pull the new person to the door with an encour-
aging gesture for them to open it (field notes, in-school phase). He was
not observed to use the doorknob himself. He knew special school doors
were locked from students' use.

The locked doors in school extended beyond a physical constraint.
Cobain had been locked into a student profile of disengagement. In his
final months at school, no one had expectations for him to be interested
in school, or its people and curriculum. He didn't "belong to the class."
This sentiment permeated engagements with his entire teaching staff, rel-
egating him to time alone with his reflection in the door.

After leaving school, Cobain's individualized programs were held in community spaces where doors were not typically locked. When not engaged in the activity at hand, which was still observed to be quite often, Cobain again spent his time by the door, as depicted in the photo on the right-hand side of Fig. 6.2. In contrast with special school, now doors held the possibility of being used for their intended purpose. Cobain knew doors within community spaces were typically unlocked, and in every observed community setting he attempted to open the doors multiple times. Consequently, support staff found ways to block or obscure the door handle.

Through this subtle gesture of trying to open doors, Cobain demonstrated knowledge about his transition. He knew what doors were for and how they were used. In the special school he didn't bother trying to open the door handle, because he knew they were locked. Yet in the community, there was now the opportunity to try.

Though at first the subtle gesture involved in (un)locked doors may seem inconsequential, when noted from a capability standpoint this change was, in fact, remarkable. First, because this gestural change went unnoticed. Certainly, staff reacted when Cobain attempted to leave an activity or premise, but this subtle shift in his awareness was only tracked, noted, and named within the scope of this research. This reflection is further compounded by the fact that, secondly, no instance was ever observed when someone explained to Cobain in a manner meaningful to him that he was finishing school. One could challenge this premise by pointing out, for example, that he attended graduation. Nonetheless, if the event was considered from Cobain's perspective, as someone with significant cognitive and sensory impairments, graduation may have been any other confusing event for which he was late and spent most of his time sitting next to someone else's family. School administration and staff did not farewell him on his final day of school. It was like any other day. It's plausible that Cobain figured out that he had transitioned from school on his own. He demonstrated this knowledge subtly through one of his preferred activities, standing by the front door.

Capability discussion (Un)locked doors are an apt symbol of potential and opportunity. In a sense, the unlocked doors of post-school community life represented Cobain's potential for freedom, no longer restricted behind the locked doors of special school. A door that is not locked could almost be seen as an invitation for future community integration. Cobain had the potential to walk through an unlocked door as much as anyone else in the community might.

Considered another way, however, Cobain's transition team may have inadvertently blocked or even intentionally re-locked the doors to his transition. Transition was a time when Cobain became absorbed and monopolized by his residential care service. His "individualized" community activities were filtered through this organization. The scene for these activities may have been set in the community, but the programs were each run by, and specifically catered only for, those within the disability care service.

A concluding question is whether Cobain's personal capabilities, such as his understanding of his transition and schedule, went unnoticed, or if were they noticed and simply ignored? It might have been too painful for his mother and others close to Cobain to acknowledge his capabilities, only to then see how restricted his transition and future opportunities had become. This line of questioning sheds light on Cobain's mother's comment about "transition being the grieving process all over again" (Quote transcription, in-school phase). A common assumption is that transition brings up emotions equivalent to that of first receiving a disability diagnosis. Perhaps emotions run even deeper, beyond the family. Another plausible component of the "grief" was a broader, societal aspect. Cobain's school years involved finding places of acceptance and support within the disability community. Attending school behind locked doors meant safety. Literal safety for students like his housemate, "the runner," as well as symbolic safety, an emotional safety net, amongst peers and families who shared similar experiences, needs, and concerns. Transition meant severing the support network of the special school. The (un)locked doors of transition open directly into the heart of community life—raw, unsheltered, unsupported, and, in many instances, not accepting. This might be why Cobain's mother positioned her son within the residential care service, so he could regain some amount of shelter. To once again lock Cobain's doors safely.

Faine Early in Faine's transition his mother said that she had always thought leaving school signaled a time when students with disability "disappear completely" (field notes, in-school phase). She had planned to retire when her son finished school so that she could be fully available for his care. After three years of special-school experiences, they were "on a new journey." Faine's mother communicated her son's impression of

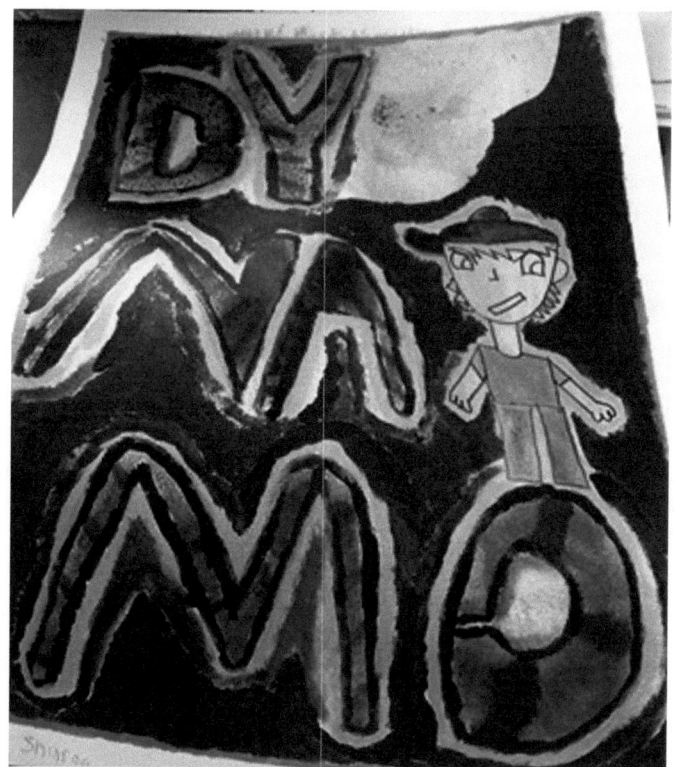

Fig. 6.3 Faine's transition metaphor: "Dynamo" drawing

special school as, "If he could stop time, it would be now. And that would be his ideal world, right now. Stop it right now" (interview transcript, Faine's mother, in-school phase). Something as good as special school was difficult to replace. She expressed a feeling of being "cheated," having not known about special school for so long, to only then have only a few year's access before aging out.

Faine was allocated enough funding to attend a community-based day program for three days each week. This was fairly common amongst his peers at the day service. He used other support funds to continue attending the community art class that was previously described. One weekday per week he spent at home.

Of his many artistic creations, Faine made a dynamo cartoon character (Fig. 6.3) drawn during his weekly community art class while he was still in school. In the drawing, the male image embodied a developing maturity akin to Faine's progression toward young adulthood. No longer a schoolboy, but without fully embracing manhood. Faine was unable to articulate these subtleties or the meaning of his word choice, "dynamo" with the text drawn in graffiti style that took over half the image. Whether by chance or by design, Faine's artwork will be described as a symbol encapsulating his educational experiences.

As previously described, Faine's family was skeptical of the public education system, and in turn, Faine's engagement with the wider community outside of his whānau family. For example, in attempts to shelter Faine, he was home-schooled for a while. Faine's mother was shaping her own life plans around preconceived unjust conditions in which her son would one day "disappear" from society altogether.

Once "found" by the special school, Faine enjoyed a great number of successes. His "dynamo" personality flourished. At age 18, it marked the first time Faine had attended a school without his mother working there as well. He flourished independently with autonomy outside of his whānau family. Faine demonstrated enormous personal capability and many interpersonal strengths in leadership.

Capability discussion Now at age 21, Faine's transition meant finding ways he could transfer his dynamo personality, and overall successes within school, to new community, post-school settings. He found this challenging, at least in part, due to his peers at the post-school day service having more significant, communication-based disabilities. By the end of research fieldwork, Faine was spending more time at home. His whānau's answer to the stresses of transition appeared to be to return Faine, once again, into their protection. This may have been their reaction to Faine's discontentment in his post-school program. His mother more than anyone saw how special school provided a place where Faine was "cherished for what he has to offer" (interview transcript, in-school phase). Yet it may be that the community offers few places for such individuals, or possibly for anyone, to feel so cherished.

Stated in capability terminology, the early stages of Faine's transition, specifically his three years at special school, expanded his capability set. He had more opportunities to meet and socialize with a diverse range of peers and participate in a variety of inclusive settings. This is not to negatively judge his youth with his mother and whānau. Rather, to note how transition had expanded opportunities he'd not experienced or considered before. Yet, after the completion of school, opportunities became restrictive and limited. Community programs and peer groups seemed less compatible with Faine's interests and priorities. He wanted more from post-school life.

USA

El Returning to El's composite narrative case transcript,

> Growing up, my parents prioritized that we traveled around the country. We did lots of road trips. I think this had a big influence on me growing up. While sitting next to my parents, I'd ask them tough questions and their answers would teach me about life. Parents always seemed to know everything.
>
> After high school I really wanted to go traveling, so I spent the next couple of years hitchhiking and riding freight trains around the country and just sightseeing. I wasn't really interested in the hitchhiking culture and that social kind of world. I was more interested in being alone and seeing beautiful places and experiencing nature in ways that you just don't really get to see by car. This was a critical turning point in my life.

El's transition metaphor is travel. Not commercial travel by plane, bus, train, or even by personal car. Rather, a bohemian style of travel that is without finance or of minimal cost, organized and executed almost entirely through personal initiative and the kindness of those who are oftentimes strangers. The hitchhiking travel format is a key distinction of El's transition symbol (Fig. 6.4). Recall that El experienced a transient childhood having little to no autonomy over the family's decisions. They moved often, frequently prompted by traumas within the family. El did not know what was going to happen next in life. In young adulthood, however, travel and the choice of the freedom of movement now became under control. Yet, interestingly, the travels that El undertook were still reliant on others. Connecting back to the earlier notion of waitlists, El continued to wait—waiting to "thumb a lift," or wait for a suitable train to slowly pass by. Such forms of travel are not solely about the destination. The focus is also on the journey.

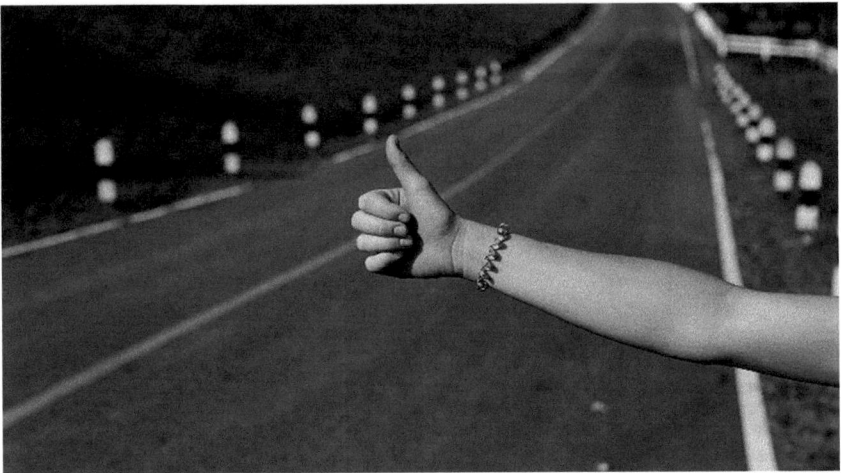

Fig. 6.4 El's transition metaphor: Travel

Capability discussion In capability terms, a key distinction of El's post-school transition is self-determinization; control over experiences that promote real freedoms outside of a dramatic childhood. More specifically, as a young adult El found a way to transform restricted resources into valuable activities and practices. Hitchhiking exemplifies a multi-variate way to promote well-being as it involves more than simply increased goods and finances. Travel of this nature is a poignant illustration of the non-materialist aspects of human well-being that are a constituent part of one's capability set. Returning to the waitlist metaphor, the value of having control over one's life experiences involves meaningful fulfillment of the passage of time (i.e., waiting) with purpose, excitement, and the thrill of future adventures. Financial goods and services, like money or better insurance coverage, would have likely moved El's name forward on the various waitlists that were restricting access to mental and physical healthcare. Yet, those alone would not have fulfilled the entire range of El's central human capabilities. Capabilities such as agency, imagination, affiliation with others, and play can be provided through the exhilaration of this style of travel.

One final note is that El traveled in this manner during the pandemic, which is no small feat. This was managed during a time when people were extremely cautious, if not legally mandated, to limit their interpersonal contacts. Yet hitching was a way that El found to "collectively reckon how we live in the world. We take care of each other." El successfully remained flexible and dynamic. Travel became an emblematic symbol of power and hope during trying times.

Dignity of Risk

One shared commonality between the cases relates to a concept known as dignity of risk. Dignity of risk was a term first used by Perske (1972) as a response to a concerning lack of access to autonomy and control over life decisions that prevented growth and development found in "experiencing the risk-taking of ordinary life" (p. 195). Reasonable risk-taking is a component part of the normalization and related deinstitutionalization movements, or the process of replacing long-stay psychiatric hospitals with less isolated community-based services. Having access to dignity of risk addresses the overprotected treatment of people with disabilities and is "part of the pathway to a full life experience. Without the power of making mistakes, individuals do not build the fortitude necessary to find success or find their start in life" (Bumble et al., 2022, p. 65).

Post-school transition for all young adults, regardless of disability, involves a known "period of floundering" that comes through the experience of, and working through, certain personal challenges (Halpern, 1985, p. 481). Therefore, dignity of risk permits young people with disabilities access to the self-esteem that develops from the right to take reasonable risks free from the cautious caregiving of others. While the term itself is not new, applications to transition are only recently emerging.

In one study, dignity of risk was assessed within inclusive post-secondary education programs. Bumble et al. (2022) identified a four-stage continuum toward dignified risk, which included (from most to least restrictive)—manufactured, programmed, managed, and authentic risk. The first stage manufactured risk within a segregated environment. For example, attending post-secondary education with a tailored curriculum held on a segregated part of campus (akin to Haku's post-school experience). Second, programmed risk, involved students giving input, say to their course of study, but required they adhere to a strict schedule for meals, study sessions, modified curriculum, etc. The third stage of managed risk involved participating in standard activities of post-secondary education. For instance, if the student completed an internship, they were provided a job coach or support assistant to meet this requirement. Lastly, authentic risk associated with the inherent risks of any post-secondary student, which might involve, for example, having a non-disabled roommate and arranging personal schedules without required check-ins. The researchers used the phrase "messy inclusion" to denote a willingness to embrace such authentic risks that might involve a wide range of discomfort, failures, and triumphs (Bumble et al., 2022, p. 66). Each were a journey during the critical stage of entering adulthood. Essentially, not all decisions need to be the "right" decision.

The benefits of experiencing authentic risk enable post-secondary students with disabilities to identify and address challenging or endangering situations. To fully identify their capabilities. Instances of dignified risk from the case narratives include: Haku taking the initiative to explore new parts of town on public transportation; Cobain discovering new spaces for leisure and relaxation as well as communication; Faine expanding his dynamic social networks beyond his whānau/family; and El's access to travel and experiencing autonomy outside of a chaotic family. All the young adult cases experienced authentic risks as described by Bumble et al. (2022) as inherent risks that anyone with or without disability might experience. Importantly, each of these transition cases extend the knowledge base beyond the setting of post-secondary education. Post-secondary education is not always a viable option for those who are more significantly impacted by disability. Yet, the availability to access a dignity of risk is an imperative component of transition nonetheless.

"A commonality of the human experience is that we know what happened yesterday but have no secure knowledge about what is going to happen tomorrow" (Garland-Thomson, 2022, p. 172). Risk is typically something that people aim to mitigate. Although dignity of risk may at first appear a simple concept, considerations are needed to address challenges that are surprisingly hard to enact, honor, and prioritize. The core of this concept involves appraisals, judgments, varying ways of knowing, evidentiary standards, and diverse definitions of risk. There also exists a central tension with the duty of care, or the responsibility to maintain the health, safety, and well-being of others. Respect for persons and their potentially risky choices also depends upon one's role within the interpersonal dynamic. Are they an educator, parent, care giver, medical professional, for instance? One illustration from within the cases was Haku's mother who was understandably concerned when her son traveled to new parts of town without forewarning. Haku's experiences would have likely differed significantly if he, like Cobain, lived within a residential care service. A balance of care responsibilities and human concerns, as well as biases or assumptions, can all impact the amount of risk afforded. Maintaining risk depends on context.

Beyond mitigation of potential hazards, dignity of risk may therefore involve addressing inequities and historical injustices, and rethinking human biases. Prospects can become limited from restricted thinking (another example of adapted preferences). With a focus on access to dignity of risk, transition becomes more than an intervention on/for students with disabilities. More than best-practice procedures. Transition becomes a human right that when done well can expand the social fabric by including people with diverse perspectives, experiences, and abilities. In this manner of thinking, promoting societal inclusiveness can benefit everyone while directly contributing to students' transition success.

Opportunity Serves Dignity

Dignified post-school transition practices can lead to a more equitable society. In addition to risk, another key feature of transition justice is the role of opportunity. Described in capability-specific language, transition "success" cannot be determined solely through one's functionings or outcomes. Transition can extend beyond outcomes-orientation, to place the unit of concern on the opportunities, or capabilities accessible to young adults with disabilities. Additionally of importance are the personal, social, and environmental conversion factors necessary to achieve priorities within one's capability set, and the freedom, choice, and agency (or dignity of risk) to implement them. When opportunities that precede the exit from school are the central unit of examination, the focus shifts to one's capability set. Essentially, what experiences are young adults having that inform, and thus precede, the implementation of their hopes, dreams, and priorities?

Trialing Trialing was a term used by some participants in ANZ as a constituent feature of transition. Despite its widespread discussion and application, the term is not explicitly used in the existing transition literature. To trial something is to test it for suitability. For example, in the ANZ narratives, this involved the selection process of post-school options while preparing to leave school. Essentially, the "doing, looking, and working it all out" of post-school community options (interview transcript, in-school phase).

Upon closer examination, each young adult case in ANZ experienced trialing that offered only a restricted range of pre-existing programs and disability-specific services. While post-school selections were made, they were chosen from a set of options so restricted, that any choice and freedom inherent within those selections were highly compromised. Individual preferences were not thoroughly considered. Rather, each young person was understood only well enough to determine which transition outcome they best suited. For instance, this was the reported logic of why Haku only trialed a post-secondary, pre-employment, education program. It was determined that he could gain employment. Were he to trial community day programs, such as the ones Cobain and Faine were exclusively shown, he might take the needed place of this often-over-enrolled option. While the transition outcomes in ANZ may have been considered successful, in some instances, insufficient consideration was given to the experiences that led up to each young adult's decisions.

In the USA case, the process of trialing was not an overt topic of discussion. It was inferred from the provided transcripts that post-school transition planning did not occur in El's case. This was likely because El never received specific services under the Individuals with Disabilities Education Act (IDEA), such as having an Individualized Education Plan (IEP). Were El to receive these services, transition planning would have begun at a maximum of age 16, or earlier in some states. Post-school goals and options would be added as a part of the IEP.

It is unclear whether El's lack of educational services was due to the family's transience, having to wait on waitlists, or some other obstacle. El was likely someone who 'slipped through the cracks' of the educational system. Yet, El was aware of certain options for mental and physical health services, as well as options for funding support. The struggle was to find help to access these services. Based on the described experiences, trialing in the USA meant less about being funneled into a disability-specific service (such as in ANZ), and more about finding and securing any access at all to services. Without having anywhere to go, El commented on being bored at home.

Capability approach is well suited to address the concerns raised in the process of trialing, which is depicted in Fig. 6.5. On the left-hand side of the figure, letters A, B, and C denote a range of pre-existing transition options. The minus symbol indicates the possibility that some combination of options may not have been trialed. Transition could essentially be

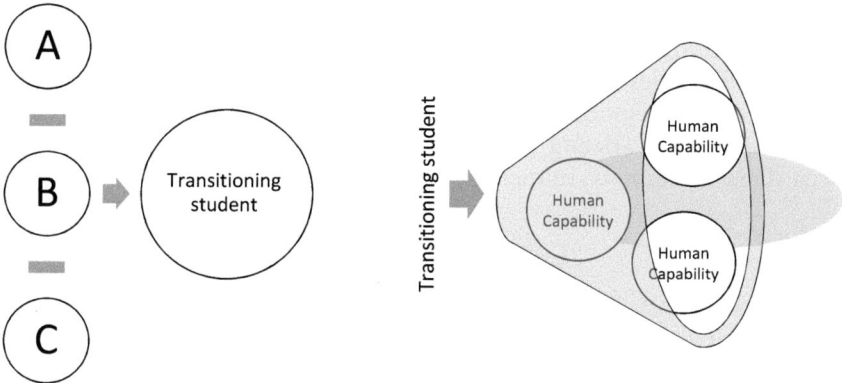

Fig. 6.5 Undignified trialing (left) and trialing with dignity (right)

procedurally completed, yet this is not the preface to a thriving post-school life.

In contrast, restructuring trialing to that of the right-hand side of Fig. 6.5 is to inform trialing through the ten human capabilities (Nussbaum, 2000). In this conception, trialing becomes the expansion of an individual's capability set through a thorough exploration of viable opportunities. This form of trialing will also signal when or where community supports are not currently available so that resources can be strategically developed as needed. For example, this may involve the need to create additional opportunities to continue intellectual pursuits (outside of formal post-secondary education), and engage with diverse peers for joy and play, as well as engage in nature with wildlife.

Returning to capability theory, trialing can be conceptualized similarly to the process of conversion from capabilities, or opportunities, to lived functionings, or the beings and doings of life. Conversion factors that bring a person from capability to lived functionings include personal choice and agency, as well as social and environmental factors. Nussbaum (2000) argued that the ten human capabilities set a standard, not for how life should turn out, but rather for what every individual should have access to, experiences that should be trialed for suitability.

Bringing the cases of ANZ and USA together, trailing based on capability can frame a new conception of transition. Nussbaum's ten human capabilities can enhance opportunities and services provided. In this manner, the priority shifts away from solely focusing on post-school outcomes, with the replacement of a full exploration of the fundamental tenets of a good life. In this alternate version of trialing, a minimum level of each of the ten capabilities would be addressed without exchanging one capability for another, or prioritizing one person's capability over, or as dependent upon, another's. Trialing practices should consider every human being, regardless of disability, in their own right.

CHAPTER CONCLUSION

The novel aspects of this work are brought together in this chapter to form a clear and distinctive understanding of a transition with dignity. The challenge is overcoming the focus on problems to consider the possibilities. Nussbaum and other moral philosophers refer to this phenomenon as adapted preferences. Namely that certain conditions are made more problematic because we expect or collude in making them be so. Much of what is known about transition for students with disability is tainted with a historical legacy of problems to which this work offers an alternative viewpoint.

When the opportunities that precede the exit from school are the central unit of examination, optimistic insights about transition arise. First, post-school transition involves a period of floundering (Halpern, 1985) that comes through the experience of, and working through, certain personal challenges. This dignity of risk permits young people with significant disabilities access to the self-esteem that develops from the right to take reasonable risks free from the cautious caregiving of others. Second, transition is more than an intervention on/for students with disabilities. A wider consideration of opportunities for societal inclusiveness can also contribute to a student's transition success or failure. Transition should be considered more than best-practice steps, but rather, as a matter of social justice. In sum, transition justice can illuminate power, privilege, and the need for international change. Special education transition research has contributed to collective knowledge on this essential topic, but expertise that exists in the lived transition experiences of individuals with significant disabilities needs not only to be understood but actioned. This work offers a window into how activating research partnerships can leverage exciting opportunities to promote change.

References

Bumble, J. L., Worth, C. R., Athamanah, L. S., Rooney-Kron, M., Regester, A., & Lidgus, J. (2022). Messy inclusion: A call for dignity of risk in inclusive post-secondary education. *Inclusive Practices, 1*(2), 64–69.

Gaffney, J. S. (2013, September). Agency in literacy learning (ALL): Possibility-driven research. In *Inaugural Professor Lecture at the Faculty of Education*. University of Auckland.

Garland-Thomson, R. (2022). What Du Bois and I know about dignity of risk. *Perspectives in Biology and Medicine, 65*(2), 171–178. https://doi.org/10.1353/pbm.2022.0012

Halpern, A. S. (1985). Transition: A look at the foundations. *Exceptional Children, 51*(6), 479–486. https://doi.org/10.1177/001440298505100604

Nussbaum, M. C. (2000). *Women and human development: The capabilities approach*. Cambridge University Press.

Nussbaum, M. C. (2006). *Frontiers of justice: Disability, nationality, species membership*. Harvard University Press.

Nussbaum, M. C. (2011). *Creating capabilities: The human development approach*. The Belknap Press.

Perske, R. (1972). The dignity of risk. In W. Wolfensberger (Ed.), *Normalization: The principle of normalization in human services* (pp. 194–200). National Institute on Mental Retardation.

CHAPTER 7

Conclusion

Abstract In this chapter, the argument is made that opportunity serves dignity. Transition can present the opportunity for each of Nussbaum's 10 capabilities to be thoroughly explored in-school and then remain viable in post-school life. This is not to say dignified outcomes must be an absolute outcome. All young adults, those with and without disabilities alike, require genuine opportunities to construct a thriving life of personal priority. Implications of a transition with dignity are here considered.

Keywords Genuine opportunity • Neurodiversity identity movement • Pandemic

GENUINE OPPORTUNITY IMPLICATIONS

As the title of the aptly named publication reminds us, there is a dignity in choice, even if it runs the risk in "people with developmental disabilities to eat too many doughnuts and take a nap" (Bannerman et al., 1990). Recall that the core of the capability approach pertains to a person's functionings, which are lived beings and doings (e.g., being well-fed or literate), and capabilities, which are the opportunities or freedoms to realize these functionings. A leap is made by the addition the qualifier *genuine*. Opportunities are genuine only insofar as they do not involve (a) undue cost or (b) risk to other functionings (Wolff & De-Shalit, 2007). In fact,

© The Author(s), under exclusive license to Springer Nature   101
Singapore Pte Ltd. 2024
S. M. Hart, *Transition with Dignity*,
https://doi.org/10.1007/978-981-97-2351-5_7

Wolff and De-Shalit prefer to use the phrase genuine opportunities to capability as a more accurate way to secure functionings.

Simply stated, people have a genuine opportunity only if the costs are reasonable, and they realistically choose a viable option they are willing to bear. To illustrate, a spouse may choose to live off their partner's income. If for some reason this spouse has been intentionally constrained from employment, then genuine opportunities are restricted. This is an interpersonal example, but restrictions may occur at individual, social, or structural levels, thus all should be considered in order for genuine opportunities to exist.

Worth consideration is whether the cases of Haku, Cobain, Faine, and El had a genuine opportunity to transition with dignity. In ANZ, opportunities were not completely genuine, because post-school options were not sufficiently trialed. Post-school goals were set without a thorough exploration of options. USA gave the impression of ingenuine opportunity because support services were not available. Reasons included not being covered by insurance, being put on waitlists, or services being costlier than welfare funding afforded. Based within these international cases of transition, a question to consider is what post-school services are truly worth (in both a financial and a non-financial sense)? Are post-school options a genuine opportunity if they are only available to a restricted few under a restricted set of circumstances?

Current restrictions in post-school programs and services means that transition procedures may actually inhibit active community engagement since genuine access is so rarely achieved. Returning to the Aesop fable, post-school options become "soured" either by lack of investigation or by lack of availability. From an adapted preferences position, any post-school option becomes better than none, or it may also be that post-school options are not worth pursuing at all. Yet, the purpose of the narrative cases in ANZ and USA were to acknowledge the inequalities, analyze the capabilities, and then to suggest new opportunities. Genuine opportunities stem from inclusion, as will be discussed in the final points about inclusive research. The responsibility for realizing flourishing life outcomes cannot be solely achieved at the interpersonal level. Social and structural changes, such as final points about the turbulent times of the pandemic, can promote practices that give all people a genuine opportunity to choose a life they have reason to value.

Vulnerability and inclusive research Vulnerability is a relative state, but is often applied to the disability experience for a predisposition to certain material, social, and emotional risks. For instance, disability status often-times correlates with an increased likelihood of poverty (material), physical abuse or hostility, such as online cyberbullying (social), or loneliness (emotional; Osgood et al., 2005). Another consideration is the way vulnerability impacts research. Vulnerable populations in research include individuals with disabilities, amongst others such as young children and those who are pregnant or incarcerated. For these groups, additional protections, considerations, and safeguards are put in place to ensure their safety from research protocols. A noted concern is that some researchers may become overburdened by these safeguards, and then opt not to include vulnerable populations within their work (Hart et al., 2020). If those with disabilities are bypassed, then their perspectives are deemed insignificant and peripheral, which results in gaps in collective knowledge. The consequences of lack of participation impede social belonging and citizenship (Taylor, 2018).

Genuine opportunity to be included in research positions those with severe and complex needs as having valuable contributions to their transitions and knowledge on this topic. Being included in research is notably different, however, from inclusive research. As such, the responsibility in this research was to take an individually tailored approach to ensure rich research participation aligned with the capabilities of each participant. Furthermore, to ensure that the implications of this work extend beyond the individual, with aims to be accessible, relevant, and empowering for the wider community sector.

Capability restrictions during pandemic times This research was conducted before and during the pandemic lockdowns. Covid can be considered a "capability crisis" (Anand et al., 2020, p. 293). During pandemic lockdowns there was a collective experience that "the positive freedoms necessary to pursue the lives people value have been constrained across the world" (p. 293). People temporarily gave up certain freedoms to protect other valued freedoms. For example, restricting body integrity of free movement for protection of bodily health. Every core element of Nussbaum's 10 central human capabilities were, and in some cases continue to be, impacted. Human connectivity has been compromised with increasing vulnerability within families, homes, and societies. Capability-limiting impacts of public health emergencies and related lockdown restrictions impact levels of depression and anxiety, as is the increasing rise in digitization that can further alienate. Inequality exist in unemployment, providing food security, and meeting the wide range of economic challenges.

Like most aspects related to the pandemic, it is hard to make sweeping statements or offer universally applicable truths. From the perspectives of school students with disabilities, there existed a range of experiences. Some had all or the majority of their support services closed. This shuttered community access brought about an upheaval in their routines. Other students had contrasting experiences. They enjoyed remote education, for instance. Accommodations long cried out for, such as online distance learning, working at a truly individualized pace, and extended one-on-one contact time with teachers became obtainable overnight (Hart, 2021).

Everyone had some experience during the pandemic that touched upon their own fragility. Holding on to these memories will help address pandemic related inequalities from a people-first perspective. Sustainable futures will develop that identify policy priorities across the range of human experience and needs. Essentially, to improve the world that young adults are leaving school to transition into. One way forward is for everyone to use their pandemic experiences to leverage their cultural preconceptions, societal assumptions, attitudes, and prejudices—filters that we take into our social encounters. Genuine opportunities can then be forged.

Conclusion A recent example from the neurodiversity autism movement is offered as a way to summarize and apply central themes to a contemporary topic. First for context, the World Health Organization estimates that worldwide about 1 in 100 children is on the autism spectrum. This is an average figure, and reported prevalence varies substantially across countries and studies. For example, Centers for Disease Control and Prevention in USA announced a pair of new reports that found 1 out of every 36 children has autism (Escher, 2023). This is a significant increase from the 2021 estimate of 1 in 44, which was then a big jump from 1 in 110 in 2006. Autism as a Spectrum of Disorders (ASD) is now more common than childhood cancer, diabetes, and AIDS combined. Furthermore, it is not fully known what causes autism. While educational and behavioral interventions exist, there is no treatment or cure. ASD does not go away, and it cannot be "grown out of." At best, it can be "grown in to" by individuals getting to know themselves over time and learning to implement adaptive strategies.

As numbers of ASD rise, so has the neurodiversity identity movement, which has gained increasing attention. The concept of neurodiversity is rooted in the disability rights movement, which states that autism is a natural variation in human experience. People interact with the world around them in many different ways, and there is no one "right" way of thinking, learning, and behaving. Neurodiversity tracks well with the distinction between the medical and social models of disability. Differences related to autism should not be viewed as deficits (or disorders as used in the classification), and should therefore be met with acceptance and support, rather than pathology or stigma. Neurodiversity has important implications for inclusivity. Contemporary examples are growing in number, from sensory-friendly community settings and events, such as sensory screenings of films that accept movement and modified noise levels, to pop-culture media such as the popular television program *The Good Doctor*.

Yet understandings about those who are more significantly impacted by disabilities are oftentimes inferred by those with less-significant disabilities. As it has been portrayed within this book, the perspectives most needing to be shared are those least able to share it. Returning to the vast spectrum of ASD, there are individuals who, for example, have little to no sense of their own personal safety and can inflict serious harm on themselves and others, even when supervised. It is questionable the extent to which the neurodiversity movement has done much to improve conditions for such individuals, those with more severe autism. In fact, it may have made matters more challenging because now certain autism-related approaches and treatments have become stigmatized. With the swelling number of those with autism who require a lifespan of care, there now exists an "epidemic of need" (Escher, 2023, para. 3).

How does this understanding of the neurodiversity identity movement apply to post-school transition? In one sense, the concept of neurodiversity is exactly what has been called for in this book. Essentially, to better transition opportunities through a more aware and accepting society. Additionally, to move away from a welfare orientation of disability in favor of human rights. Yet, when considered through the lens of capability there are a few cautions in the balance. The first caution is that the medical and social models within the neurodiversity movement are likely insufficient standing on their own in binary opposition. Capability portrays the multifaceted complexity and diversity of the disability experience by including matters of race, culture, and economics, to name just a few. A multidimensional variety of individually tailored supports and community developments need to be more insistently advocated. The next caution is neurodiversity has placed an imbalanced spotlight on some more than others, as for instance popular media tends to portrays autism as akin to a super power. Those who are less informed may make false assumptions and correlations between those who experiences autism in vastly different ways. Lastly, the pace of future treatments, services, and possibly even a cure, might decelerate as a response to neurodiversity advocacy. The neurodiversity movement has positively moved the needle for disability advocacy, but should equally serve as an important reminder to ensure genuine opportunities to a diverse range of disability experiences.

Broadly speaking, genuine opportunities mean a life worthy of dignity for every human being, those with and without disability alike. The focus is on human flourishing. Thriving rather than merely surviving. An awareness of human rights that are so real and essential that they may at times be taken for granted. Expanded opportunities within the transition of young adults with significant disabilities and those who support them, may in turn improve a thriving life for all.

References

Anand, P., Ferrer, B., Gao, Q., Nogales, R., & Unterhalter, E. (2020). COVID-19 as a capability crisis: Using the capability framework to understand policy challenges. *Journal of Human Development and Capabilities, 21*(3), 293–299. https://doi.org/10.1080/19452829.2020.1789079

Bannerman, D. J., Sheldon, J. B., Sherman, J. A., & Harchik, A. E. (1990). Balancing the right to habilitation with the right to personal liberties: The rights of people with developmental disabilities to eat too many doughnuts and take a nap. *Journal of Applied Behavior Analysis, 23*(1), 79–89. https://doi.org/10.1901/jaba.1990.23-79

Escher, J. (2023). *The autism surge: Lies, conspiracies, and my own kids.* The Free Press.

Hart, S. M. (September 2021). *Diverse voices on disability advocacy during the pandemic in the US. Breaking Boundaries – (Counter) Accounts during the Pandemic.* Open Access Collection.

Hart, S. M., Pascucci, M., Sood, S., & Barrett, E. M. (2020). Value, vulnerability and voice: An integrative review on research assent. *British Journal of Learning Disabilities, 48*(2), 154–161. https://doi.org/10.1111/bld.12309

Osgood, W., Foster, E. M., Flanagan, C., & Ruth, G. R. (2005). *On your own without a net: The transition to adulthood for vulnerable populations.* University of Chicago Press.

Taylor, A. (2018). Knowledge citizens? Intellectual disability and the production of social meanings within educational research. *Harvard Educational Review*, *88*(1), 1–25. https://doi.org/10.17763/1943-5045-88.1.1

Wolff, J., & De-Shalit, A. (2007). *Disadvantage*. Oxford University Press. https://doi.org/10.1093/acprof:oso/9780199278268.003.0005

REFERENCES

Albrecht, G. L. (1973). Socialization in the rehabilitation process. *Health Services Research, 8*(1), 67.

Alverson, C. Y., Lindstrom, L. E., & Hirano, K. A. (2019). High school to college: Transition experiences of young adults with autism. *Focus on Autism and Other Developmental Disabilities, 34*(1), 52–64. https://doi.org/10.1177/1088357615611880

Anand, P., Ferrer, B., Gao, Q., Nogales, R., & Unterhalter, E. (2020). COVID-19 as a capability crisis: Using the capability framework to understand policy challenges. *Journal of Human Development and Capabilities, 21*(3), 293–299. https://doi.org/10.1080/19452829.2020.1789079

Aron, L., & Loprest, P. (2012). Disability and the education system. *The Future of Children, 22*(1), 97–122. https://www.jstor.org/stable/41475648

Bannerman, D. J., Sheldon, J. B., Sherman, J. A., & Harchik, A. E. (1990). Balancing the right to habilitation with the right to personal liberties: The rights of people with developmental disabilities to eat too many doughnuts and take a nap. *Journal of Applied Behavior Analysis, 23*(1), 79–89. https://doi.org/10.1901/jaba.1990.23-79

Barton, L. (2005). Emancipatory research and disabled people: Some observations and questions. *Educational Review, 57*(3), 317–327. https://doi.org/10.1080/00131910500149325

Belich, J. (2001). *Paradise reforged: A history of the New Zealanders from 1880 to the Year 2000.* Penguin Books.

Bengtsson, M. (2016). How to plan and perform a qualitative study using content analysis. *Nursing Plus Open, 2*, 8–14. https://doi.org/10.1016/j.npls.2016.01.001

Bigby, C., Frawley, P., & Ramcharan, P. (2014). Conceptualizing inclusive research with people with intellectual disability. *Journal of Applied Research in Intellectual Disabilities, 27*, 3–12. https://doi.org/10.1111/jar.12083

Brantlinger, E., Jimenez, R., Klingner, J., Pugach, M., & Richardson, V. (2005). Qualitative studies in special education. *Exceptional Children, 71*(2), 195–207. https://doi.org/10.1177/001440290507100205

Bumble, J. L., Worth, C. R., Athamanah, L. S., Rooney-Kron, M., Regester, A., & Lidgus, J. (2022). Messy inclusion: A call for dignity of risk in inclusive post-secondary education. *Inclusive Practices, 1*(2), 64–69.

Carter, E. W., Brock, M. E., & Trainor, A. A. (2014). Transition assessment and planning for youth with severe intellectual and developmental disabilities. *The Journal of Special Education, 47*(4), 245–255. https://doi.org/10.1177/0022466912456241

Carter, E. W., Awsumb, J. M., Schutz, M. A., & McMillan, E. D. (2021). Preparing youth for the world of work: Educator perspectives on pre-employment transition services. *Career Development and Transition for Exceptional Individuals, 44*(3), 161–173. https://doi.org/10.1177/2165143420938663

Certo, N. J., Luecking, R. G., Murphy, S., Brown, L., Courey, S., & Belanger, D. (2008). Seamless transition and long-term support for individuals with severe intellectual disabilities. *Research and Practice for Persons with Severe Disabilities, 33*(3), 85–95. https://doi.org/10.2511/rpsd.33.3.85

Creese, J., Byrne, J. P., Conway, E., Barrett, E., Prihodova, L., & Humphries, N. (2021). "We all really need to just take a breath": Composite narratives of hospital doctors' well-being during the COVID-19 pandemic. *International Journal of Environmental Research and Public Health, 18*(4), 2051–2069. https://doi.org/10.3390/ijerph18042051

Dalkilic, M., & Vadeboncoeur, J. A. (2016). Re-framing inclusive education through the capability approach: An elaboration of the model of relational inclusion. *Global Education Review, 3*(3).

Davies, M. D., & Beamish, W. (2009). Transitions from school for young adults with intellectual disability: Parental perspectives on "life as an adjustment". *Journal of Intellectual and Developmental Disability, 34*(3), 248–257. https://doi.org/10.1080/13668250903103676

Deardorff, M. E., Pulos, J. M., Suk, A. L., Williams-Diehm, K. L., & McConnell, A. E. (2020). What do transition assessments look like for students with a significant cognitive disability? A multistate survey of educational stakeholders. *Inclusion, 8*(1), 74–85. https://doi.org/10.1352/2326-6988-8.1.74

Denzin, N. K. (2001). *Interpretive interactionism* (2nd ed.). Sage.

Django, P. (2021). Culturally sustaining pedagogies and our futures. *The Educational Forum*, *85*(4), 364–376. https://doi.org/10.1080/0013172 5.2021.1957634

Escher, J. (2023). *The autism surge: Lies, conspiracies, and my own kids*. The Free Press.

Forber-Pratt, A. J. (2020). Musings from the streets of India: Voice for the disabled who are nonverbal. *Qualitative Inquiry*, *26*(7), 827–832. https://doi.org/10.1177/1077800419846635

Gaffney, J. S. (2013, September). Agency in literacy learning (ALL): Possibility-driven research. In *Inaugural Professor Lecture at the Faculty of Education*. University of Auckland.

Gaffney, J. S., Morton, M., & Hart, S. M. (2017). Aotearoa New Zealand. In J. Patton & M. Wehmeyer (Eds.), *Handbook of international special education* (Vol. 3). Santa Barbara, CA.

Garland-Thomson, R. (2022). What Du Bois and I know about dignity of risk. *Perspectives in Biology and Medicine*, *65*(2), 171–178. https://doi.org/10.1353/pbm.2022.0012

Halpern, A. S. (1985). Transition: A look at the foundations. *Exceptional Children*, *51*(6), 479–486. https://doi.org/10.1177/001440298505100604

Hart, S. M. (September 2021). Diverse voices on disability advocacy during the pandemic in the US. *Breaking Boundaries – (Counter) Accounts during the Pandemic*. Open Access Collection.

Hart, S. M. (2022). Agentic ethnography: Methods, positionality, and perspectives of individuals with significant disabilities on the transition from school. *International Journal of Research and Method in Education*, *45*(1), 3–17. https://doi.org/10.1080/1743727X.2021.1881057

Hart, S. M., Hill, M. F., & Gaffney, J. S. (2015). Teachers absent: Impacts upon the transition of students with significant special needs. In D. Garbett & A. Ovens (Eds.), *Teaching for tomorrow today* (pp. 491–498). Edify.

Hart, S. M., Gaffney, J. S., & Hill, M. F. (2017). Critical reflections on emancipatory partnerships in transition research: Discerning perspectives of New Zealand Students on the autism spectrum. *Disability and Society*, *32*(6), 831–852. https://doi.org/10.1080/09687599.2017.1329710

Hart, S. M., Gaffney, J. S., & Hill, M. F. (2019). Opportunity to transition with dignity: Silos and trialing in Aotearoa New Zealand. *Canadian Journal of Children's Rights / Revue canadienne des droits des enfants*. Themed issue on Disability and Children's Rights. *6*(1). doi:https://doi.org/10.22215/cjcr.v6i1.2124.

Hart, S. M., Pascucci, M., Sood, S., & Barrett, E. M. (2020). Value, vulnerability and voice: An integrative review on research assent. *British Journal of Learning Disabilities*, *48*(2), 154–161. https://doi.org/10.1111/bld.12309

Hart, S. M., Hill, M. F., & Gaffney, J. S. (2021). Timetabling a transition with dignity: Perspectives of young adults with significant support needs. *Journal of Intellectual and Developmental Disability, 46*(3), 227–238. https://doi.org/1 0.3109/13668250.2021.1885973

Hetherington, S. A., Durant-Jones, L., Johnson, K., Nolan, K., Smith, E., Taylor-Brown, S., & Tuttle, J. (2010). The lived experiences of adolescents with disabilities and their parents in transition planning. *Focus on Autism and Other Developmental Disabilities, 25*(3), 163–172. https://doi.org/10.1177/1088357610373760

Hopper, K. (2007). Rethinking social recovery in schizophrenia: What a capabilities approach might offer. *Social Science and Medicine, 65*(5), 868–879. https://doi.org/10.1016/j.socscimed.2007.04.012

Institute of Education Sciences, National Center for Special Education Research (1989). *National longitudinal transition study.* Author: Retrieved from: https://nces.ed.gov/pubsearch/pubsinfo.asp?pubid=NCEE20154014

Institute of Education Sciences, National Center for Special Education Research (2009). *National longitudinal transition study-2.* Author: Retrieved from: https://ies.ed.gov/ncser/projects/nlts2/

Johnston, O., Wildy, H., & Shand, J. (2023). Student voices that resonate: Constructing composite narratives that represent students' classroom experiences. *Qualitative Research, 23*(1), 108–124. https://doi.org/10.1177/14687941211016158

Lakoff, G., & Johnson, M. (2008). *Metaphors we live by.* University of Chicago Press.

Mazzotti, V. L., Rowe, D. A., Kwiatek, S., Voggt, A., Chang, W.-H., Fowler, C. H., Poppen, M., Sinclair, J., & Test, D. W. (2021). Secondary transition predictors of postschool success: An update to the research base. *Career Development and Transition for Exceptional Individuals, 44*(1), 47–64. https://doi.org/10.1177/2165143420959793

McCoy, S., Shevlin, M., & Rose, R. (2020). Secondary school transition for students with special educational needs in Ireland. *European Journal of Special Needs Education, 35*(2), 154–170. https://doi.org/10.1080/08856257.2019.1628338

Miles, M., & Huberman, A. M. (1994). *Qualitative data analysis: An expanded sourcebook* (2nd ed.). Sage.

Ministry of Education. (2023). *Education in New Zealand: Our education system.* Author. Retrieved from: https://www.education.govt.nz/our-work/our-role-and-our-people/education-in-nz/

Mitra, S. (2006). The capability approach and disability. *Journal of Disability Policy Studies, 16*(4), 236–247. https://doi.org/10.1177/10442073060160040501

Mitra, S., & Ruger, J. P. (Eds.). (2019). *Health, disability, and the capability approach.* Routledge.

Mutua, K., & Smith, R. M. (2006). Disrupting normalcy and the practical concerns of classroom teachers. In S. Danforth & S. L. Gabel (Eds.), *Vital questions facing disability studies in education* (1st ed., pp. 121–132). Lang.

Myers, F., Ager, A., Kerr, P., & Myles, S. (1998). Outside looking in? Studies of the community integration of people with learning disabilities. *Disability and Society, 13*(3), 389–413. https://doi.org/10.1080/09687599826704

Newman, L. A, Wagner, M., Knokey, A., Marder, C., Nagle, K., Shaver, D., Wei, X., Cameto, R., Contreras, E., Ferguson, K., Greenes, S., & Schwarting, M. (2011). *The post-high school outcomes of young adults with disabilities up to 8 years after high school. A report from the National Longitudinal Transition Study-2 (NLTS2) (NCSER 2011—3005).* U. S. Department of Education. https://files.eric.ed.gov/fulltext/ ED524044.pdf

Noblit, G. W., & Hare, R. D. (1988). *Meta-ethnography: Synthesizing qualitative studies.* Qualitative research methods series (Vol. 11). Sage.

Nussbaum, M. C. (2000). *Women and human development: The capabilities approach.* Cambridge University Press.

Nussbaum, M. C. (2006). *Frontiers of justice: Disability, nationality, species membership.* Harvard University Press.

Nussbaum, M. C. (2011). *Creating capabilities: The human development approach.* The Belknap Press.

Office for Disability Issues. (2023). *Disability action plan 2019 – 2023.* Retrieved from: https://www.odi.govt.nz/disability-action-plan-2/

Office of Special Education and Rehabilitative Services, United States Department of Education. (2020). *A transition guide: To postsecondary education and employment for students and youth with disabilities.* District of Columbia.

Organisation for Economic Co-operation and Development. (2022). *Education at a glance: Education GPS.* Paris. Retrieved from: https://www.oecd.org/education/education-at-a-glance/

Osgood, W., Foster, E. M., Flanagan, C., & Ruth, G. R. (2005). *On your own without a net: The transition to adulthood for vulnerable populations.* University of Chicago Press.

Paris, D. (2021). Culturally sustaining pedagogies and our futures. *The Educational Forum, 85*(4), 364–376. https://doi.org/10.1080/00131725.2021.1957634

Perske, R. (1972). The dignity of risk. In W. Wolfensberger (Ed.), *Normalization: The principle of normalization in human services* (pp. 194–200). National Institute on Mental Retardation.

Plotner, A. J., Mazzotti, V. L., Rose, C. A., & Teasley, K. (2020). Perceptions of interagency collaboration: Relationships between secondary transition roles, communication, and collaboration. *Remedial and Special Education, 41*(1), 28–39. https://doi.org/10.1177/0741932518778029

Robeyns, I. (2021). *Wellbeing, freedom, and social justice: The capability approach re-examined.* Open Book Publishers. Retrieved from: https://socialsci.libretexts.org/Bookshelves/Sociology/Cultural_Sociology_and_Social_Problems/Wellbeing_Freedom_and_Social_Justice%3A_The_Capability_Approach_Re-Examined_(Robeyns)

Scheef, A., & Mahfouz, J. (2020). Supporting the post-school goals of youth with disabilities through use of a transition coordinator. *Research in Educational Administration and Leadership, 5*(1), 43–69. https://doi.org/10.30828/real/2020.1.2

Schutt, R. K. (2018). *Investigating the social world: The process and practice of research.* Sage.

Seale, J., Nind, M., & Parsons, S. (2014). Inclusive research in education: Contributions to method and debate. *International Journal of Research and Method in Education, 37*(4), 347–356. https://doi.org/10.1080/1743727X.2014.935272

Sen, A. (1999). *Development as freedom.* Oxford University Press.

Shakespeare, T. (2018). *Disability: The basics.* Routledge.

Shogren, K. A., & Wehmeyer, M. L. (2020). *Handbook of adolescent transition education for youth with disabilities* (2nd ed.). Routledge.

Sitlington, P. L., Neubert, D. A., & Clark, G. M. (2010). *Transition education and services for students with disabilities* (5th ed.). Pearson.

Smith, S. R. (2013). Citizenship and disability: Incommensurable lives and well-being. *Critical Review of International Social and Political Philosophy, 16*(3), 403–420. https://doi.org/10.1080/13698230.2013.795708

Smith, P., & Routel, C. (2010). Transition failure: The cultural bias of self-determination and the journey to adulthood for people with disabilities. *Disability Studies Quarterly, 30*(1).

Taylor, A. (2018). Knowledge citizens? Intellectual disability and the production of social meanings within educational research. *Harvard Educational Review, 88*(1), 1–25. https://doi.org/10.17763/1943-5045-88.1.1

Test, D. W., Mazzotti, V. L., Mustian, A. L., Fowler, C. H., Kortering, L. J., & Kohler, P. H. (2009). Evidence based secondary transition predictors for improving postschool outcomes for students with disabilities. *Career Development for Exceptional Individuals, 32*, 160–181. https://doi.org/10.1177/0885728809346960

The White House. (2023). *Our Government.* District of Columbia. Retrieved from: https://www.whitehouse.gov/about-the-white-house/our-government/.

Trainor, A. A. (2017). *Transition by design: Improving equity and outcomes for adolescents with disabilities.* Teachers College Press.

Trainor, A. A., Newman, L., Garcia, E., Woodley, H. H., Traxler, R. E., & Deschene, D. N. (2019). Postsecondary education-focused transition planning experiences of English learners with disabilities. *Career Development and Transition for Exceptional Individuals*, 42(1), 43–55. https://doi.org/10.1177/2165143418811830

Trainor, A. A., Carter, E. W., Karpur, A., Martin, J. E., Mazzotti, V. L., Morningstar, M. E., & Rojewski, J. W. (2020). A framework for research in transition: Identifying important areas and intersections for future study. *Career Development and Transition for Exceptional Individuals*, 43(1), 5–17. https://doi.org/10.1177/21651434198645

Transparency International. (2022). *Corruption perceptions index*. Berlin. Retrieved from: https://www.transparency.org/en/cpi/2022

United Nations. (2023). *Human Development Index (HDI)*. Published online at OurWorldInData.org. Retrieved from: https://ourworldindata.org/human-development-index

United Nations General Assembly. (2007). *Convention on the rights of persons with disabilities: Resolution adopted by the General Assembly*. Retrieved from http://www.refworld.org/docid/45f973632.html

Valle, J. W., & Connor, D. J. (2019). *Rethinking disability: A disability studies approach to inclusive practices*. Routledge.

Ward, L., & Townsley, R. (2005). 'It's about a dialogue...' Working with people with learning difficulties to develop accessible information. *British Journal of Learning Disabilities*, 33(2), 59–64. https://doi.org/10.1111/j.1468-3156.2005.00346.x

Wehmeyer, M., & Patton, J. (2017). *Handbook of international special education*. Praeger.

Whaikaha, Ministry of Disabled People. (2023). *Who we are*. Wellington. Retrieved from: https://www.whaikaha.govt.nz/about-us/who-we-are/

Willis, R. (2019). The use of composite narratives to present interview findings. *Qualitative Research*, 19(4), 471–480. https://doi.org/10.1177/1468794118787711

Wolff, J. (2009). Cognitive disability in a society of equals. *Metaphilosophy*, 40(3-4), 402–415. https://doi.org/10.1111/j.1467-9973.2009.01598.x

Wolff, J., & De-Shalit, A. (2007). *Disadvantage*. Oxford University Press. https://doi.org/10.1093/acprof:oso/9780199278268.003.0005

INDEX

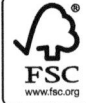